O A P N
OXFORD AMERICAN POCKET NOTES

HIV and Cardiovascular Risk

This material is not intended to be, and should not be considered, a substitute for medical or other professional advice. Treatment for the conditions described in this material is highly dependent on the individual circumstances. While this material is designed to offer accurate information with respect to the subject matter covered and to be current as of the time it was written, research and knowledge about medical and health issues is constantly evolving, and dose schedules for medications are being revised continually, with new side effects recognized and accounted for regularly. Readers must therefore always check the product information and clinical procedures with the most up-to-date published product information and data sheets provided by the manufacturers and the most recent codes of conduct and safety regulation. Oxford University Press and the authors make no representations or warranties to readers, express or implied, as to the accuracy or completeness of this material, including without limitation that they make no representations or warranties as to the accuracy or efficacy of the drug dosages mentioned in the material. The authors and the publishers do not accept, and expressly disclaim, any responsibility for any liability, loss, or risk that may be claimed or incurred as a consequence of the use and/or application of any of the contents of this material.

The Publisher is responsible for author selection and the Publisher and the Author(s) make all editorial decisions, including decisions regarding content. The Publisher and the Author(s) are not responsible for any product information added to this publication by companies purchasing copies of it for distribution to clinicians.

Disclosures

Dr. Glesby has no current relationships to disclose. In the past he has served as a consultant for and received grants and research support from Serono Laboratories.

O A P N
OXFORD AMERICAN POCKET NOTES

HIV and Cardiovascular Risk

By

Marshall J. Glesby, MD, PhD
Associate Professor of Medicine and Public Health
Division of Infectious Diseases
Department of Medicine
Weill Cornell Medical College
Regional Clinical Director, New York-New Jersey
AIDS Education and Training Center
New York, New York

OXFORD
UNIVERSITY PRESS

OXFORD
UNIVERSITY PRESS

Oxford University Press, Inc., publishes works that further
Oxford University's objective of excellence
in research, scholarship, and education.

Oxford New York

Auckland Cape Town Dar es Salaam Hong Kong Karachi
Kuala Lumpur Madrid Melbourne Mexico City Nairobi
New Delhi Shanghai Taipei Toronto

With offices in
Argentina Austria Brazil Chile Czech Republic France Greece
Guatemala Hungary Italy Japan Poland Portugal Singapore
South Korea Switzerland Thailand Turkey Ukraine Vietnam

Copyright © 2011 by Oxford University Press, Inc.

Published by Oxford University Press, Inc.
198 Madison Avenue, New York, New York 10016
www.oup.com

Oxford is a registered trademark of Oxford University Press

All rights reserved. No part of this publication may be reproduced,
stored in a retrieval system, or transmitted, in any form or by any
means, electronic, mechanical, photocopying, recording, or
otherwise, without the prior permission of Oxford University Press.

ISBN: 978-0-19-973730-7

9 8 7 6 5 4 3 2 1
Printed in the United States of America
on acid-free paper

TABLE OF CONTENTS

1 Introduction 1

2 Coronary Heart Disease 1

Epidemiology 1

Pathogenesis 2

Diagnosis and Evaluation 13

Management of Risk Factors 14

Management of Coronary Heart Disease 31

3 Dilated Cardiomyopathy 31

Epidemiology 31

Pathology/Pathogenesis 32

Diagnosis and Management 33

4 Primary Pulmonary Hypertension 34

Epidemiology 34

Pathogenesis 34

Diagnosis and Management 35

5 Pericardial Disease 36

Epidemiology 36

Pathogenesis 36

Diagnosis and Management 38

6 Endocarditis 39

Epidemiology 39

7 Cardiac Tumors 39
8 Conduction Abnormalities 40
9 Clinician Resources 42
10 Patient Resources 42
   References 43

HIV AND CARDIOVASCULAR RISK

INTRODUCTION

Mortality rates from acquired immune deficiency syndrome (AIDS)-related complications have decreased dramatically with the advent of potent, combination antiretroviral therapy. Recent data from Denmark based on mortality rates from 2000 to 2005 suggest that an average 25-year-old infected with human immunodeficiency virus (HIV) may be expected to live for another four decades,[1] approaching the lifespan of the general population. This dramatic prolongation of life has also raised the specter of increasing morbidity and mortality in the HIV-infected population related to diseases typically associated with increasing age, including cardiovascular disease (CVD). In the current HIV treatment era, leading causes of mortality include end-stage liver disease attributable primarily to co-infection with hepatitis C virus, malignancies, and cardiovascular disease.[2-4] Given these trends, clinicians caring for HIV-infected patients must be familiar with the spectrum of CVD in this population.

This book is organized by type of CVD, weighted in proportion to the epidemiologic importance in the HIV-infected population. The emphasis is on the unique issues facing the HIV-infected patient. When management does not differ in this population, the reader is referred to other sources for general management considerations.

CORONARY HEART DISEASE

Epidemiology

Shortly after the advent of combination, protease inhibitor–based antiretroviral therapy, case reports of myocardial infarction (MI) among relatively young HIV-infected patients raised concern about the potential for accelerated atherosclerosis in this population.[5,6] Subsequently, multiple analyses from cohort studies, clinical and administrative databases, and the occasional clinical trial have provided consistent evidence that the risk of MI or hospitalization for coronary heart disease (CHD) is increased in HIV-infected patients relative to HIV-uninfected patients. The magnitude of this increased relative risk is in the range of 1.5–2.5 across most of these studies.[7–11] Importantly, the absolute risk of coronary events has been relatively low in these studies to date, presumably due to the relatively young age of participants in most studies. For example, in the Data Collection on Adverse Effects of Anti-HIV Drugs (D:A:D) study, a compilation of 11 cohorts of HIV-infected patients, predominantly from Europe, with 94,469 person-years of observation, the overall rate of MI was 3.65 per 1000 person-years of observation.[12] Rates of coronary events have not increased over time in the DAD study, perhaps due to more aggressive risk-factor reduction, such as treatment of dyslipidemia and smoking cessation.[13,14]

Pathogenesis

The pathogenesis of CHD in the HIV-infected patient is likely complex and multifactorial. Conceptually, being HIV infected may be associated with increased CHD risk through mechanisms related to the infection itself or through antiretroviral therapy, each of which could affect risk directly or indirectly by altering traditional risk factors (see Figure 1). For many of the potential contributing risk factors discussed

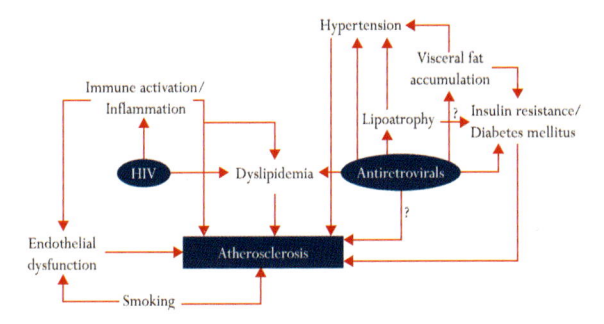

Figure 1 Pathogenesis of Atheroscelorosis in the HIV-Infected Patient.

here, both HIV infection and antiretroviral therapy likely play pathogenetic roles. Furthermore, HIV infection may be a marker of being part of a population with an increased prevalence of traditional risk factors not related to HIV or its therapy, such as smoking.[15]

Dyslipidemia

Uncontrolled, advanced HIV disease is associated with low levels of total cholesterol, high-density lipoprotein cholesterol (HDL-C), and low-density lipoprotein cholesterol (LDL-C) but high levels of triglycerides.[16,17] Despite the overall low LDL-C concentration, the proportion of atherogenic small, dense LDL-C may be increased.[18] With treatment of HIV, LDL-C often increases, perhaps in large part due to improved health and nutritional status rather than direct effects of antiretrovirals on LDL-C metabolism.[19,20]

Most contemporary initial antiretroviral regimens consist of two nucleoside reverse transcriptase inhibitors (NRTIs) plus either a non-nucleoside reverse transcriptase inhibitor (NNRTI) or protease inhibitor (PI). The PI is most often combined with a low dose of ritonavir, a PI used to inhibit cytochrome P450-based metabolism of the active PI to boost its levels. There are multiple drugs within each of these three classes (Table 1), and treatment guidelines often list preferred and alternative options within each class based on efficacy and safety concerns.[21,22] Some clinicians use an integrase inhibitor instead of an NNRTI or PI as the third agent in an initial regimen.[23] When resistance to specific antiretrovirals is present at baseline or develops over time due to incomplete virologic suppression, treatment options may be constrained.

Table 1 Antiretroviral Drugs
Nucleoside Reverse Transcriptase Inhibitors
• Abacavir • Didanosine • Emtricitabine • Lamivudine • Stavudine • Tenofovir* • Zidovudine
Non-Nucleoside Reverse Transcriptase Inhibitors
• Delavirdine • Efavirenz • Nevirapine • Etravirine

Table 1 Continued
Protease Inhibitors
- Atazanavir
- Darunavir
- Fosamprenavir
- Indinavir
- Lopinavir/ritonavir
- Nelfinavir
- Ritonavir
- Saquinavir
- Tipranavir
Fusion Inhibitor
- Enfuvirtide
CCR5 Inhibitor
- Maraviroc
Integrase Inhibitor
- Raltegravir
Co-Formulated Antiretrovirals**
- Abacavir/lamivudine
- Tenofovir/emtricitabine
- Tenofovir/emtricitabine/efavirenz
- Zidovudine/lamivudine
- Zidovudine/lamivudine/abacavir
*Tenofovir is a nucleotide reverse transcriptase inhibitor
**Lopinavir/ritonavir is listed under protease inhibitors

The effects of antiretroviral therapy on lipids are complicated to assess and summarize due to the concurrent use of multiple drugs in individual patients. In most studies, it is difficult to separate the effects of suppressing HIV replication, improving overall health status, and potential direct effects of antiretrovirals on lipids. A few studies of the short-term administration of specific drugs to healthy HIV-uninfected volunteers provide some insights into the direct effects of the drugs on lipid metabolism, but these data are limited. Some general differences exist between classes of antiretrovirals, as well as between drugs within each class; nonetheless, several generalizations can be made:

- Within the NRTI class, stavudine appears to have adverse effects on LDL-C and triglycerides, possibly due to mitochondrial toxicity.[24] Tenofovir, a nucleotide analog in common use, may actually lower non-HDL-C (i.e., total cholesterol minus HDL-C, a readily calculated parameter that contains the major atherogenic lipoproteins).[25] Other commonly used drugs, such as lamivudine, emtricitabine, and abacavir appear to be relatively neutral.[26–28]

- Several of the NNRTI drugs appear to favorably increase HDL-C by an unknown mechanism. Efavirenz, the most commonly used drug in this class, may also increase triglycerides and non–HDL-C more so than nevirapine.[29] The favorable effects of efavirenz on HDL-C, however, generally result in minimal change in the total cholesterol-to-HDL-C ratio, suggesting that the net effect on CHD risk is neutral.[20,29] Delavirdine, a now seldom-used NNRTI, is also associated with increases in HDL-C.[30] Etravirine, an NNRTI that may retain activity against HIV that is resistant to other available NNRTIs, however, does not appear to increase HDL-C.[31]

- Most PIs appear to cause triglyceride elevations, especially when boosted with low-dose ritonavir. Atazanavir, when given without ritonavir, does not adversely affect lipids; the addition of low-dose ritonavir to atazanavir results in modest increases in triglycerides and LDL-C.[32] Fos-amprenavir administered without ritonavir also appears to be neutral with regard to lipids.[33] In clinical trials of most contemporary ritonavir-boosted PI regimens, HDL-C has typically increased.[34-36] LDL-C increases have been more variable.

- Maraviroc, an HIV entry inhibitor that blocks the major HIV co-receptor, CCR5, and raltegravir, an integrase inhibitor that blocks integration of HIV into the host cell's DNA, both appear to be neutral with regard to lipids.[37,38] The effects of enfuvirtide, an HIV fusion inhibitor, on lipids are difficult to assess since it has been studied almost exclusively in highly treatment-experienced patients who have added other drugs to their regimens in addition to enfuvirtide.[39]

Antiretroviral therapy may also contribute to CHD risk independent of its effects on lipids. In the DAD study, the relative risk of MI was 1.16 per year of exposure to combination antiretroviral therapy, which was attributable to use of PI-, rather than NNRTI-based therapy.[12] Adjustment for changes in lipids over time, however, did not completely attenuate the association between PI use and MI, suggesting that factors other than adverse effects on lipids also contribute to this relationship.

Recent data have also found associations between the use of specific antiretrovirals and MI. Recent use of abacavir and didanosine were associated with increased risk of MI in the DAD observational cohort study, and the association with abacavir was corroborated in the Strategies for the Management of Antiretroviral Therapy (SMART) study.[40,41]

Other analyses of clinical trials and cohort studies, however, have not found an association between abacavir use and MI.[42-44] Some of the cohort studies have adjusted for concurrent CHD risk factors to address channeling bias, whereby patients with underlying risk factors may be preferentially prescribed abacavir given its neutral effects on lipids, although such adjustment may be imperfect. Along these lines, lack of adjustment for renal insufficiency in some studies, which might lead to preferential prescribing of abacavir rather than the potentially nephrotoxic drug tenofovir, could also account for the association between abacavir and MI.[44] Renal insufficiency, including even mild impairment, is associated with increased risk of MI and CHD death in the general population.[45-47] No proven biologic mechanism links abacavir to CHD risk, although some have postulated proinflammatory effects and/or adverse effects on platelet aggregation or endothelial function, although data are inconclusive to date.[48,49]

In summary, data from observational cohorts and clinical trials are somewhat inconsistent and inconclusive with regard to associations between specific antiretrovirals and CHD events. The underlying risk of CHD should be considered when selecting antiretroviral regimens, and action should be taken to minimize all modifiable risk factors (e.g., hypertension, dyslipidemia, diabetes mellitus, and smoking). Clinicians should consider the effects of individual antiretrovirals on lipids and potential associations with CHD, including those that may emerge in future studies, when designing antiretroviral regimens for patients with underlying CHD risk factors.

HIV AND CARDIOVASCULAR RISK

Inflammation

Inflammation plays an important role in the pathogenesis of atherosclerosis.

HIV infection is a proinflammatory state, especially when viral replication is unchecked. Recent data from the SMART study highlight the potential importance of uncontrolled viral replication in the pathogenesis of CHD in HIV-infected patients. This study randomized both antiretroviral naïve and experienced patients to intermittent CD4-cell–guided therapy versus continuous therapy. Patients in the intermittent therapy arm cycled on and off antiretrovirals when their CD4 cell counts crossed thresholds of less than 250 cells/mm^3 for starting and greater than 350 cells/mm^3 for stopping. The trial was stopped prematurely due to excess morbidity and mortality in the intermittent therapy arm.[50] Of note, there were more CHD events (defined as nonfatal MI, silent MI, nonfatal stroke, coronary artery disease requiring surgery, or death from cardiovascular disease) in the intermittent therapy versus the continuous therapy arm (1.3 vs. 0.8 per 100 person-years; $P = 0.05$). The total cholesterol-to-HDL-C ratio increased during treatment interruption, which may have contributed to CHD risk.[51] Perhaps more plausibly, the acute relationship between treatment interruption and CHD events may be due to increased inflammation related to unopposed viral replication. Indeed, overall mortality in SMART was linked to d-dimer and interleukin (IL)-6 levels.[52]

Even patients with HIV viral loads below the level of detection may have ongoing immune activation and inflammation that could contribute to atherosclerosis. For example, so-called elite controllers—HIV-infected patients with undetectable

HIV viral loads in the absence of antiretroviral therapy—have increased carotid intima-medial thickness relative to HIV-uninfected controls.[53] Several studies have examined the effects of antiretroviral therapy on high-sensitivity C-reactive protein (hsCRP),[36,54,55] an acute phase reactant that is predictive of CHD events in the general population, independent of traditional risk factors. The results of these studies are conflicting, but provide no compelling evidence that hsCRP decreases substantially as a result of suppressing HIV replication. Recent analysis of an administrative database suggests that hsCRP may be predictive of CHD in HIV-infected patients.[56] Others have found an association between the magnitude of cytomegalovirus-specific CD8+ T-cell responses and the degree of carotid intima-medial thickness in HIV-infected patients.[57] Data are conflicting as to whether HCV co-infection is associated with CHD in HIV-infected patients.[58,59]

Disordered Glucose Metabolism

Insulin resistance and diabetes mellitus are well established risk factors for CHD, and both may be more prevalent in HIV-infected patients. Data are conflicting on whether HIV-infected patients are at increased risk of diabetes mellitus,[60,61] but insulin resistance is likely more common in this population.[62] The pathogenesis of insulin resistance is likely multifactorial, with potential contributions from antiretrovirals, hepatitis C virus co-infection, altered fat distribution, and traditional risk factors (see Figure 2). Cumulative exposure to NRTIs is associated with insulin resistance and incident diabetes,[60,63,64] possibly due to mitochondrial toxicity.[65,66] Certain protease inhibitors, such as

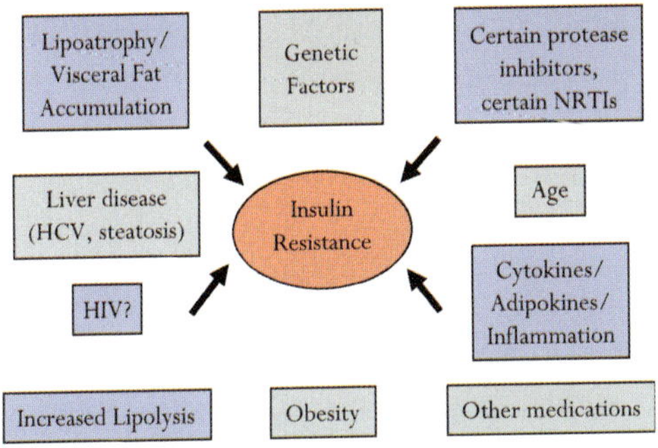

Figure 2 Factors That May Contribute to Insulin Resistance in HIV-Infected Patients.

---

the now seldom-used drug indinavir, can induce measurable insulin resistance in healthy volunteers, likely due to inhibition of the Glut-4 glucose transporter.[67,68]

Altered Fat Distribution

Shortly after the advent of potent, combination antiretroviral therapy, investigators began to report altered fat distribution in HIV-infected patients, often termed *lipodystrophy*. Initial reports documented loss of subcutaneous fat (lipoatrophy) most prominently in the face, extremities, and buttocks with concurrent gain of visceral abdominal fat (lipoaccumulation), sometimes with accompanying dorsocervical fat pad enlargement.[69–71] Subsequent careful epidemiologic studies with HIV-uninfected controls have demonstrated that, although lipoatrophy is uniquely seen in HIV-infected patients, abdominal fat accumulation is not more common on average in this population.[72–74] Clinical experience, however, suggests that a subset of HIV-infected patients has significant lipoaccumulation.

These changes in fat distribution have been linked to dyslipidemia and insulin resistance, suggesting that afflicted patients often have a form of metabolic syndrome.[75] In particular, patients with lipoatrophy are sometimes very insulin resistant,[76] perhaps related to diminished capacity to store circulating free fatty acids.[77]

Lipoatrophy has been linked specifically to use of thymidine analog NRTIs (stavudine more so than zidovudine) and is likely a manifestation of mitochondrial toxicity.[78-81] Mitochondrial dysfunction could theoretically contribute to atherogenesis via oxidative stress or other mechanisms. Limiting the use of thymidine analogs will likely reduce the incidence of lipoatrophy. Lipoaccumulation is more vexing in that its pathogenesis is not understood.

Hypertension

There are very few rigorously performed studies of blood pressure in the HIV-infected population. The prevalence of hypertension does not appear to be increased in HIV-infected patients compared to the general population.[82,83] Data are conflicting on whether blood pressure increases after initiation of antiretroviral therapy.[84-86] Incident hypertension has been linked more often to traditional risk factors rather than to specific antiretrovirals,[87] although associations have been reported anecdotally between indinavir use and hypertension.[88,89] Weight gain and changes in fat distribution, both lipoatrophy and lipoaccumulation, are also associated with elevated blood pressure.[75,90,91] HIV-associated nephropathy, which is seen almost exclusively in patients of African descent, and other forms of renal disease may cause hypertension in the HIV population.[92,93]

Endothelial Dysfunction

Endothelial dysfunction is thought to be important in the initiation of atherosclerosis. Uncontrolled HIV viremia, dyslipidemia, insulin resistance, immune dysfunction, and specific antiretrovirals, such as indinavir, have been linked to endothelial dysfunction in the HIV population.[94–97]

Lifestyle Factors

Multiple studies have documented a high prevalence of smoking among HIV-infected populations, with ranges of 35–72%.[98] While these high rates may be attributable largely to demographic and socioeconomic factors that are also linked to HIV acquisition, the high prevalence of depression in HIV-infected patients may also contribute. In the current HIV treatment era, obesity has overtaken wasting as the major weight-related issue in populations with access to antiretrovirals.[99] Cocaine and crystal methamphetamine use may also contribute to CHD events in HIV-infected patients.[100–102]

Diagnosis and Evaluation

The diagnosis of CHD does not differ in HIV-infected patients compared to the general population. There is no clear role for screening tests, such as exercise stress tests, in asymptomatic individuals. Consensus panels have recommended checking fasting lipid profiles (total cholesterol, triglycerides, HDL-C, and calculated LDL-C) in HIV-infected patients prior to initiating antiretroviral therapy, approximately 3–6 months thereafter, and then annually in stable patients.[103,104] Patients with baseline triglyceride elevations should have lipids checked within a month or two after starting antiretrovirals that may adversely affect triglycerides (e.g., ritonavir-boosted PI, efavirenz). In the setting of triglyceride elevations above 400 mg/dL, the calculated LDL-C from a standard lipid panel derived using the Friedewald equation is inaccurate. Simply calculating the non–HDL-C is a useful proxy measure of CHD risk in the setting of significant hypertriglyceridemia. Directly measuring LDL-C is a less readily available alternative and poses additional cost, and the accuracy of some clinically available assays may be suboptimal relative to the gold standard of ultracentrifugation.[105] Given the potential for increased risk of diabetes mellitus, clinicians should monitor fasting glucose levels along with lipids.[104] The role of checking other biomarkers, such as hsCRP or d-dimer, is more controversial and not validated in this population. It may be reasonable to assess hsCRP to further risk-stratify select patients found to be at intermediate risk of CHD in order to determine how aggressively to intervene with risk factor reduction.

Management of Risk Factors

Controversy exists over the risk–benefit profile of aspirin for primary prevention of vascular disease in the general population.[106,107] No data are available on the use of aspirin for the primary prevention of CHD in HIV-infected patients with cardiac risk factors.

Smoking

Smoking cessation is the one intervention likely to have the greatest effect on reduction of CHD events. Nonetheless, specific data in HIV-infected patients are limited.[108,109] Data are also limited on drug interactions between smoking cessation agents and antiretrovirals. A short-term interaction study in healthy volunteers found a minimal effect of low-dose ritonavir on bupropion exposure, the latter of which is metabolized primarily by cytochrome P450 2B6.[110] In contrast, lopinavir/ritonavir decreased exposure to bupropion and its active metabolite by approximately 50% in another study of healthy volunteers, suggesting that higher doses of bupropion may be needed when these drugs are co-administered.[111] Data are nonetheless insufficient to recommend specific dose adjustment. Given high rates of psychiatric comorbidities in HIV-infected patients, clinicians should use bupropion and varenicline cautiously, since each has been associated with adverse psychiatric effects.[112]

Dyslipidemia

Consensus guidelines recommend adapting the National Cholesterol Education Program Adult Treatment Panel III (NCEP ATP III) approach to dyslipidemia for HIV-infected patients, in which the intensity of risk-reduction therapy is based on the patient's risk of a CHD event.[103,113]

Patients with diabetes mellitus, known CHD, or other atherosclerotic disease are considered to be at high risk (>20% predicted risk of MI or cardiac death over 10 years). Whether HIV itself should be considered a risk-equivalent state akin to diabetes mellitus is controversial. Clinicians should risk-stratify patients as per the algorithm in Figure 3 by adding up the number of major CHD risk factors and

Patient Assessment

- Instruct patient to fast for 9–12 hours (may take medications with water).
- Check fasting lipid panel (total cholesterol, HDL-C, TGs, calculated LDL-C*) prior to starting antiretroviral regimen and 3-6 months after.
  - *If TG > 400 mg/dL, calculated LDL-C is not reliable.
    Calculate non-HDL-C = Total cholesterol – HDL-C, or, send directly measured LDL-C.
  - If TG ≥ 200 mg/dL calculate non-HDL-C, which is a secondary goal of therapy after LDL-C.
- Consider secondary causes of dyslipidemia (e.g., hypothyroidism, nephrotic syndrome, excessive alcohol intake, medication-induced [e.g., thiazides, testosterone], poorly controlled diabetes mellitus)
- Risk stratify

Does patient have established coronary heart disease (CHD)?
Does patient have a coronary risk equivalent (1 or more of the following)?
- ☐ Cerebrovascular disease   ☐ Abdominal aortic aneurysm
- ☐ Peripheral vascular disease   ☐ Diabetes mellitus

No — Count CHD risk factors

Yes — High risk category

① Current CHD Risk Factors:
check all that apply
- ☐ Cigarette smoking
- ☐ Hypertension (BP ≥140/90 or on antihypertensive medication)
- ☐ Age (men ≥ 45, women > 55 years)
- ☐ Family history of premature CHD
  - √ In male first-degree relative < 55 years
  - √ In female first-degree relative < 65 years
- ☐ Low HDL-C (< 40 mg/dL)*
  *Subtract one risk factor if HDL-C > 60 mg/dL.

② Number of Risk Factors:
- ≥ 2: Calculate 10-year risk of CHD event using Framingham calculator
- 0–1 : low risk

(http://hin.nhlbi.nih.gov/atpiii/calculator.asp) or see Framingham Calculator Worksheets

③ Risk Categories
- If risk > 20%, patient has coronary risk equivalent state
- 10–20% moderate risk
- < 10% lower risk

Figure 3 Management of Dyslipidemia and HIV: Patient Assessment.

This tool was developed by the Lipid Disorders subset (Chair: Marshall Glesby, MD, NY/NJ AETC) of the AIDS Education and Training Centers (AETC) National Resource Center: Primary Care Management for the HIV/AIDS Provider Workgroup (Chair: Jerey Beal, MD, FL/Caribbean AETC). Collaborating members include Daniel Lee, MD (Pacific AETC), Laura Armas, MD (TX/OK AETC), Carl Fitchtenbaum, MD (Pennsylvania/MidAtlantic AETC) and Pamela Rothpletz-Puglia (AETC NRC). The workgroup reports were coordinated by the AETC National Resource Center (Managing Editor: Rianna Stefanakis), 2008.

HIV AND CARDIOVASCULAR RISK

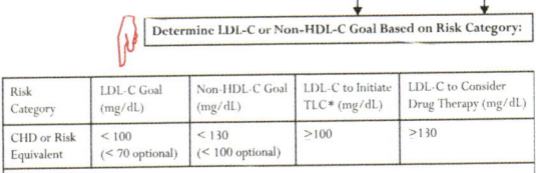

Determine LDL-C or Non-HDL-C Goal Based on Risk Category:

Risk Category	LDL-C Goal (mg/dL)	Non-HDL-C Goal (mg/dL)	LDL-C to Initiate TLC* (mg/dL)	LDL-C to Consider Drug Therapy (mg/dL)
CHD or Risk Equivalent	< 100 (< 70 optional)	< 130 (< 100 optional)	>100	>130
≥2 risk factors and 10-yr risk:				
10–20%	< 130 (< 100 optional)	< 160 (< 130 optional)	>130	>130
<10%	< 130	< 160	>130	>160
0-1 risk factor	< 160	< 190	>160	>190

* TLC = Therapeutic Lifestyle Change

Figure 3 Continued.

calculating the Framingham risk score for those with two or more risk factors (see Figure 4). Data from the DAD study indicate that the observed number of cardiac events is similar to the number predicted by the Framingham equation.[114] Investigators are trying to develop HIV-specific risk calculators but until one is available, it is appropriate to use the Framingham calculator, which is available for download (see Clinician Tools).

As in the general population, LDL-C is the primary target for most HIV-infected patients at risk for CHD, and non–HDL-C is a secondary target in those with hypertriglyceridemia. The non–HDL-C goal is simply the LDL-C goal plus 30 mg/dL. While elevations in both LDL-C and triglycerides may coexist in HIV-infected patients, isolated low HDL-C or low HDL-C with hypertriglyceridemia are quite common.[115]

Framingham Point Scores
Estimate of 10-year Risk

Men

STEP 1. Calculate the number of points for each risk factor.

AGE

Age	Points
20-34	-9
35-39	-4
40-44	0
45-49	3
50-54	6
55-59	8
60-64	10
65-69	11
70-74	12
75-79	13

TOTAL CHOLESTEROL†

mg/dL	20-39	40-49	50-59	60-69	70-79
<160	0	0	0	0	0
160-199	4	3	2	1	0
200-239	7	5	3	1	0
240-279	9	6	4	2	1
≥280	11	8	5	3	1

SMOKING*

Age	20-39	40-49	50-59	60-69	70-79
Non-Smoker	0	0	0	0	0
Smoker	8	5	3	1	1

HDL†

mg/dL	Points
>60	-1
50-59	0
40-49	1
<40	2

SYSTOLIC BLOOD PRESSURE‡

mm Hg	untreated	treated
<120	0	0
120-129	0	1
130-139	1	2
140-159	1	2
≥160	2	3

STEP 2. Sum the points for each risk factor. The 10-year risk for myocardial infarction and coronary death (hard CHD) is estimated from total points, and the person is categorized according to absolute 10-year risk.

TOTAL POINTS	<0	0	1	2	3	4	5	6	7	8	9	10	11	12	13	14	15	16	≥17
10-YR RISK, %	<1	1	1	1	1	1	2	2	3	4	5	6	8	10	12	16	20	25	≥30

HIV AND CARDIOVASCULAR RISK

Women

AGE	STEP 1. Calculate the number of points for each risk factor.							
	TOTAL CHOLESTEROL[1] Age				SMOKING* Age	HDL[†]	SYSTOLIC BLOOD PRESSURE	
Age	Points	mg/dL	20–39 40–49 50–59 60–69 70–79		20–39 40–49 50–59 60–69 70–79	mg/dL	mm Hg untreated	treated

Figure 4 Management of Dyslipidemia and HIV: Framington Point Scores.

This tool was developed by the Lipid Disorders subset (Chair: Marshall Glesby, MD, NY/NJ AETC) of the AIDS Education and Training Centers (AETC) National Resource Center: Primary Care Management for the HIV/AIDS Provider Workgroup (Chair: Jerey Beal, MD, FL/Caribbean AETC), Collaborating members include Daniel Lee, MD (Pacific AETC), Laura Armas, MD (TX/OK AETC), Carl Fitchtenbaum, MD (Pennsylvania/MidAtlantic AETC) and Pamela Rothpletz-Puglia (AETC NRC). The workgroup reports were coordinated by the AETC National Resource Center (Managing Editor: Rianna Stefanakis), 2008.

Lifestyle modification is an important first step in the management of dyslipidemia in the HIV-infected patient, as in the general population (Table 2). Patients should be counseled to engage in regular aerobic activity, ideally at least 30 minutes per day on most, if not all, days of the week.[116] Excess consumption of saturated fats is common in HIV-infected patients, and associated with hypertriglyceridemia.[117] Reducing alcohol consumption may help hypertriglyceridemia.[118] Dietary counseling should include a reduction in saturated fats to less than 7% of calories and a cholesterol intake of less than 200 mg/d.[118] Referral to a dietician can be helpful in this regard. There are few rigorous studies of the effects of lifestyle modification on dyslipidemia in the HIV population, but the available

Table 2 Lifestyle Interventions for Dyslipidemia
Hypercholeseterolemia
• Reduce intake of saturated and trans fats to < 7% of calories
• Reduce intake of dietary cholesterol to < 200 mg per day
• Plant stanols/sterols: 2 g/day
• Viscous (soluble) fiber: 10-25 g/day
• Supplement with almonds, soy
Hypertriglyceridemia
• Restrict saturated and trans fats
• Emphasize omega-3 and monounsaturated fats
• Limit simple carbohydrates
• Restrict alcohol
• Exercise
• Weight loss
Adapted from: NCEP ATP III. JAMA. 2001;285:2486-2497

data suggest that triglycerides are more responsive than cholesterol.[119,120]

If patients are not at targeted lipid levels after a 4-8-week trial of lifestyle intervention, pharmacologic lipid-lowering therapy may be necessary. Alternatively, modifying antiretroviral therapy may be an option for some patients. The advantages and disadvantages of each approach are summarized in (Table 3).

One randomized clinical trial suggested that lipid-lowering therapy with pravastatin or bezafibrate (a drug similar to

---

Table 3 Advantages of Lipid-Lowering Therapy versus Changing Antiretroviral Regimens

Advantages of Lipid-Lowering Therapy

- Proven clinical benefit in the general population for some drugs (e.g., statins)
- Potential pleiotropic effects beyond LDL-C reduction (e.g., anti-inflammatory effects, plaque stabilization from statins)
- Limited data suggest greater efficacy compared with switching antiretrovirals
- Avoids potential adverse effects of new antiretroviral regimen
- Avoids risk of loss of virologic suppression and emergence of resistance to a new antiretroviral regimen

Advantages of Changing Antiretroviral Therapy

- Avoid pill burden and cost of additional medications
- Avoid potential drug interactions with lipid-lowering agents
- Avoid potential toxicities of lipid-lowering agents

fenofibrate) resulted in greater reductions in lipids compared to switching a PI to efavirenz or nevirapine.[121] In general, it is difficult to attribute LDL-C elevations to a specific antiretroviral drug, making switching antiretroviral therapy a less attractive alternative. In contrast, if severe hypertriglyceridemia develops after initiation of a ritonavir-boosted PI, for example, it may be reasonable to consider switching antiretrovirals. The most important consideration is maintenance of virologic suppression. Clinicians must consider the individual's treatment history and resistance pattern, if known, before contemplating a change in antiretroviral therapy. Randomized, controlled data support the short-term safety and efficacy of several types of antiretroviral switches for managing dyslipidemia:

- PI to NNRTI[121,122]
- Ritonavir-boosted or unboosted PI to atazanavir[123,124]
- Thymidine analog NRTI (stavudine or zidovudine) to tenofovir or abacavir[125]

A recent randomized trial of switching from lopinavir/ritonavir to raltegravir (an integrase inhibitor) resulted in decreased total cholesterol, triglycerides, and non–HDL-C.[126] The study, however, failed to show noninferiority of raltegravir to continuing lopinavir/ritonavir with regard to maintaining HIV virologic suppression. The enrollment of some patients with extensive prior antiretroviral experience and presumed resistance to the NRTI components of their regimens may have contributed to this finding. Switching a ritonavir-boosted PI to raltegravir is a potential strategy for managing dyslipidemia only if the NRTI backbone is fully active, such as in the setting of an initial antiretroviral regimen with no prior treatment failure.

Similar considerations apply to initiating antiretroviral therapy in patients with dyslipidemia at baseline or those with multiple CHD risk factors. In this setting, regimens that do not adversely affect lipids are preferable.[127]

The basic approach to pharmacologic management of dyslipidemia depends on whether LDL-C or non–HDL-C is the predominant problem versus severe hypertriglyceridemia (>500 mg/dL) (see Figure 5).

Statins are the mainstay of managing LDL-C elevations. Clinically significant drug–drug interactions occur between statins and both PIs and NNRTIs (Table 4).[128–131] Co-administration of simvastatin and lovastatin with PIs is contraindicated, as the concentration of the statin may increase dramatically and cause toxicity[128]; there is one anecdotal report of a death due to such an interaction.[132] A more modest interaction occurs with atorvastatin, which can be used safely at low doses with PIs.[128] Rosuvastatin levels nearly double when co-administered with lopinavir/ritonavir, yet the lipid-lowering activity appears to be attenuated.[131] Clinical experience suggests that low-dose rosuvastatin can probably be used safely with lopinavir/ritonavir with caution; limited data are available with other PIs. Pravastatin has been used widely in HIV-infected patients, since its levels tend to be reduced with most PIs,[129,133,134] with the exception of darunavir, where levels are increased by about

Patient Management

- Address non-lipid risk factors (e.g., smoking cessation, treating hypertension)
- Recommend lifestyle changes; refer to dietician if possible. Encourage aerobic exercise (30–60 mins >5 times/week).
- Reassess lipids in 4–8 weeks.
- If high LDL-C or TGs are deemed related to HAART, consider changing antiretrovirals if treatment history permits. Examples:
  - Switching within PI class (e.g., to atazanavir with or without low dose ritonavir) or from PI to NNRTI
  - Switching d4T to alternative NRTI such as tenofovir or abacavir

If not at lipid goals at 4–8 weeks, consider pharmacologic lipid-lowering therapy

↓

Lipid-Lowering Therapy

↑LDL-C or ↑ non-HDL-C and TG < 500 mg/dL

Check baseline LFTs and creatine kinase (CK) level before initiating lipid lowering therapy. Transaminase levels > 3x upper limit of normal are a relative contraindication for statin use. Asymptomatic CK elevations are common and useful to document at baseline but are not a contraindication for statin use. Start statin[1]:

- Pravastatin 20–40 mg daily

OR

- Atorvastatin 10 mg daily

OR

- Rosuvastatin 5–10 mg daily

OR

- Fluvastatin 20–40 mg daily

Monitor:
- Check LFTs and fasting lipids in 4–6 weeks.
- Monitor LFTs at least every 6 monts thereafter[2]

Further dosage guidelines:

Titrate up dose of statin as tolerated to reach lipid goal, checking fasting lipids and LFTs after 4–6 weeks of dose change.
- **Pravastatin:** Maximum recommended dose 80 mg daily
- **Atorvastatin:** Maximum recommended dose 80 mg daily
- **Rosuvastatin:** Maximum recommended dose 40 mg daily (10 mg if on lopinavir/ritonavir)
- **Fluvastatin:** Maximum recommended dose 80 mg daily

Routine monitoring of creatine kinase in asymptomatic patients is not recommended. Myalgias with normal CK are frequently reported and may respond to switching to an alternative statin. Discontinue statin for muscle symptoms and CK > 10 x upper limit of normal. Be aware of uncommon but serious side effect of rhabdomyolysis.[*]

TG ≥500 mg/dL[3]

Start fibrate:
- Gemfibrozil 600 mg bid (before breakfast and dinner)

OR

- Micronized fenofibrate 48–145 mg daily

Alternatives:
- Fish oil capsules (2–4 g/day omega-3 fatty acids [EPA + DHA[4]])
- Check fasting lipids and LFTs in 4–6 weeks

If TGs remain ≥500:
- Reinforce diet/exercise
- Consider adding fish oil or referral to lipid specialist

HIV AND CARDIOVASCULAR RISK

> **If LDL-C/non-HDL-C remains high:** Consider adding ezetimibe 10 mg daily or extended release niacin (starting dose 500 mg at bedtime) and may titrate up to 2000 mg at bedtime) or refer to lipid specialist.
>
> Note: Incidence of cutaneous flushing and hepatoxicity are reduced with extended release formulations of niacin (e.g., Niaspan®).

Rhabdomyolysis: *

Symptoms:
- Dark, red, or cola colored urine is the hallmark along with muscle pain, weakness, or tenderness
- Fever, nausea, and vomiting may also occur

Diagnosis:
- Urinalysis may reveal casts and may be positive for hemoglobin in the absence of RBC on microscopic exam
- Positive urine or serum myoglobin
- High creatine kinase (CK, CPK)
- Serum potassium may be high

Hospitalization and aggressive management may be indicated.

Footnotes:

1. Simvastatin, pravastatin and atorvastatin levels are reduced with concomitant therapy with efavirenz or nevirapine. Pravastatin levels are reduced with the use of ritonavir or nelfinavir. Pravastatin levels are increased with the use of darunavir/ritonavir, with some individuals having up to 10-fold elevations in pravastatin exposure. Pending the availability of further data, co-administration of pravastatin and darunavir/ritonavir should be avoided. Simvastatin and lovastatin are contraindicated if patient is taking cytochrome P450 inhibitors (e.g., PIs, delavirdine). Atorvastatin levels are increased modestly with concurrent use of cytochrome P450 inhibitors; consider maximum dose of 40 mg daily in presence of such inhibitors. Rosuvastatin levels are increased with the use of lopinavir/ritonavir, though lipid-lowering efficacy may be diminished. The maximum recommended dose of rosuvastatin is 10 mg daily when used with lopinavir/ritonavir. Data on rosuvastatin in HIV-infected patients are limited.

2. For ALT (SGPT) or AST (SGOT) > 3 to 5 times the upper limit of normal, consider dose reduction, interruption, or discontinuation of statin.

3. Lowering of TGs may unmask elevated LDL-C. If high TGs and high LDL-C co-exist, consider combination therapy with fenofibrate + statin, which is associated with increased risk of rhabdomyolysis.

Non-HDL-C is a secondary target of therapy when TGs are high. Non-HDL-C lowering may be achieved by intensifying LDL-C lowering or adding niacin or a fibrate.

4 EPA = eicosapentaenoic acid

DHA = docosahexaenoic acid. Add the amounts of the long chain omega-3 fatty acids EPA plus DHA listed on the label of the fish oil supplement to determine the number of grams/day; 1000 mg = 1 gram.

Figure 5 Management of Dyslipidemia and HIV: Patient Management.

This tool was developed by the Lipid Disorders subset (Chair: Marshall Glesby, MD, NY/NJ AETC) of the AIDS Education and Training Centers (AETC) National Resource Center: Primary Care Management for the HIV/AIDS Provider Workgroup (Chair: Jerey Beal, MD, FL/Caribbean AETC), Collaborating members include Daniel Lee, MD (Pacific AETC), Laura Armas, MD (TX/OK AETC), Carl Fitchenbaum, MD (Pennsylvania/MidAtlantic AETC) and Pamela Rothpletz-Puglia (AETC NRC). The workgroup reports were coordinated by the AETC National Resource Center (Managing Editor: Rianna Stefanakis), 2008.

Table 4 Drug Interactions Between Lipid-Lowering Drugs and Protease Inhibitors or Delavirdine

Significant Interaction – Concurrent Use Contraindicated	Moderate Interaction – Initiate at Low Dose	Low Potential for Interaction
Lovastatin[128]	Atorvastatin[128]	Fluvastatin
Simvastatin[128]	Rosuvastatin[131]	Pravastatin[128,129]* Ezetimibe Fibrates Fish oil Niacin

*Co-administration of darunavir with pravastatin increases pravastatin exposure and is contraindicated.[130]

80%.[130] The prescribing information for darunavir considers concurrent use of pravastatin to be contraindicated.[135]

Bile acid sequestrants (e.g., cholestyramine, colestipol, colesevelam) should not be used, in general, as their effects on antiretroviral absorption are unknown and they may exacerbate preexisting hypertriglyceridemia.

Co-administration of efavirenz, and by extension other NNRTIs, leads to reduced levels of atorvastatin, pravastatin, and simvastatin.[136] Consequently, higher doses of statins may be needed when given with NNRTIs, with the exception of delavirdine, which likely inhibits rather than induces the metabolism of statins. Clinicians should pay particular attention to patients taking a statin who switch from NNRTI- to PI-based regimens, as the potential for toxicity exists if the statin dose is not adjusted downward with this transition.

Clinicians should monitor liver enzymes periodically in patients on statins. While a baseline serum creatine kinase level may be useful in the event that the patient develops myalgias, routine monitoring of creatine kinase is not recommended. Patients who develop myalgias on one statin sometimes tolerate a different statin.

When hypertriglyceridemia predominates, there are several treatment options, each with limited data in the HIV population. Among the fibrates, both gemfibrozil and fenofibrate are safe and efficacious at lowering triglycerides.[134,137] Extended-release niacin effectively lowered triglycerides and non–HDL-C in two uncontrolled pilot studies in HIV-infected patients.[138,139] Modest adverse effects on insulin sensitivity were seen in both studies of niacin in HIV-infected patients, the clinical significance of which is unclear given that the drug can be used safely in diabetics. The dose of extended-release niacin should be titrated upward from a starting dose of 500 mg at bedtime at 4-week intervals as tolerated to a maximal dose of 2,000 mg/d. Premedication with aspirin 30 minutes prior to dosing and use of an extended-release formulation of niacin reduces the incidence of flushing. Fish oil is another potential option with short-term safety and efficacy data from several clinical trials.[140–142] The dose of fish oil supplements should be 2 to 4 g/day of the sum of the docosahexaenoic acid (DHA) plus eicosapentaenoic acid (EPA) components.

One Food and Drug Administration (FDA)-approved fish oil supplement is currently available. As a general principle, LDL-C typically increases when triglycerides are lowered.[134]

Clinicians may need to consider combination lipid-lowering therapy in patients who do not respond adequately to monotherapy. There are limited HIV-specific data on pravastatin plus fenofibrate[134] and fenofibrate plus fish oil[141] that demonstrate short-term safety and additional benefit from adding the second agent. The incidence of muscle toxicity may be increased when combining a statin and fibrate. Fenofibrate may have a lower incidence of myopathy than gemfibrozil when used concurrently with statins.[143] There are no data on niacin plus a statin, which may be a useful combination for some HIV-infected patients. Controlled data demonstrate that the addition of ezetimibe, a cholesterol absorption inhibitor, to a statin provides further LDL-C lowering.[144] Controversy exists, however, about whether, in the general population, LDL-C lowering by ezetimibe has clinical benefit since its addition to simvastatin did not affect progression of carotid intima-medial thickness in patients with familial hypercholesterolemia.[145] Unexpectedly, there was a higher incidence of cancer in the ezetimibe arm of a placebo-controlled trial of add-on therapy to simvastatin in patients with aortic stenosis.[146] An analysis of data from two other trials of ezetimibe, however, did not find evidence to support an increased risk of malignancy.[147] Pending the availability of more definitive data, clinicians should consider ezetimibe judiciously and limit its use to scenarios where significant LDL-C elevations persist despite maximal statin doses or when statin dose escalation is limited by tolerability.

HIV AND CARDIOVASCULAR RISK

Disordered Glucose Metabolism

The management of diabetes mellitus in the HIV-infected patient is similar to that in the general population with a few caveats. If hyperglycemia or diabetes develops soon after starting a PI, it is reasonable to try switching the PI to an alternative agent or to a PI that is not known to induce insulin resistance, if the HIV treatment history permits. Metformin has been used safely in HIV-infected patients on NRTIs[148-151] despite initial concerns about the potential for lactic acidosis, which is a class effect of NRTIs that rarely occurs absent the use of stavudine and didanosine.[152-154] Recent data suggest that hemoglobin A1c values may underestimate glycemia in HIV-infected patients, related to macrocytosis (mean corpuscular volume elevations) and use of NRTIs, especially abacavir.[155] If fasting glucose values or patient records of fingerstick values suggest that the hemoglobin A1c is inappropriately low, fructosamine levels could be used to monitor glycemic control. Fructosamine levels reflect glycemic control over the preceding 2–3 weeks.[156]

Impaired fasting glucose (values of 100–125 mg/dL) and impaired glucose tolerance (2-hour glucose value 140–199 mg/dL on a 75 g oral glucose tolerance test) are both relatively common in HIV-infected patients when looked for.[157] Lifestyle interventions are appropriate, including modest weight loss (5–10% of body weight), moderate-intensity exercise (30 minutes daily), and smoking cessation.[158] Metformin therapy could be considered in this setting based on efficacy data from the general population.[159]

Hypertension

The management of hypertension in the HIV-infected patient is similar to that in the general population. Lifestyle intervention is appropriate and includes weight loss if indicated, increasing physical activity, moderating alcohol consumption, and restricting dietary sodium. When pharmacologic therapy is indicated, clinicians should be aware of potential interactions between PIs and both β-blockers and calcium channel antagonists.[160] If drugs in these classes are used, they should be started at low doses, with careful dose titration based on response and potential toxicities. Similar caution applies to losartan.[161]

Lipoaccumulation

Interventions to reduce visceral abdominal fat accumulation have the potential to reduce CHD risk since waist circumference is associated with CHD in the general population.[162,163] Furthermore, interventions that reduce visceral fat may also have favorable effects on other associated risk factors.[164,165] Aerobic exercise has been shown to reduce abdominal fat and improve lipid profiles in several small studies of HIV-infected patients and is the treatment of choice.[166,167] Most randomized switch studies of antiretrovirals have not had beneficial effects on abdominal fat.[168] Metformin may be a useful adjuvant to exercise in diabetic or pre-diabetic patients with intact renal and hepatic function, although it may exacerbate coexisting lipoatrophy.[149,169,170] Tesamorelin, an investigational recombinant human growth hormone releasing hormone analog, is promising as a short-term intervention. In a placebo-controlled trial, tesamorelin given by subcutaneous injection reduced visceral abdominal fat by 15% and the total to HDL cholesterol ratio by approximately one-third.[165]

Lipoatrophy

Although often considered primarily a cosmetic issue, lipoatrophy is frequently associated with significant insulin resistance.[76] Using research tools to monitor results, switching from a thymidine analog (stavudine or zidovudine) to an alternative NRTI, such as tenofovir or abacavir, has resulted in demonstrable gains in limb fat, although such gains may not always be noticeable to patients.[125,171–173] Thiazolidinedione drugs have also been studied as off-label treatments of lipoatrophy with mixed results.[174–176]

Management of Coronary Heart Disease

The management of established CHD does not differ in HIV-infected patients, and a detailed discussion of this topic is beyond the scope of this book. Of note, limited data suggest that rates of coronary artery, stent, or bypass graft reocclusion after revascularization procedures may be increased in HIV-infected patients.[177–179]

DILATED CARDIOMYOPATHY

Epidemiology

In the era prior to the availability of potent combination antiretroviral therapy, the prevalence of dilated cardiomyopathy in HIV-infected patients from autopsy and echocardiographic studies ranged from 10% to 30%.[180]

Cardiomyopathy has been associated with advanced HIV disease and lower CD4 cell counts, and is independently associated with death.[181] In a small case series published in 1994, about half of HIV-infected patients with cardiomyopathy had evidence of myocarditis.[182] The epidemiology of dilated cardiomyopathy in the current HIV treatment era is not well characterized, although clinical experience suggests that it is now less common; ongoing cohort studies will be informative.[183,184] Limited data suggest that left ventricular diastolic dysfunction may now be more common than systolic dysfunction.[185,186]

Pathology/Pathogenesis

Multiple potential factors can cause myocardial dysfunction in HIV-infected patients. HIV can directly infect cardiac myocytes, albeit at a low frequency.[187] Transgenic mice expressing noninfectious HIV *tat* protein develop cardiomyopathy with evidence of mitochondrial damage.[188] Other indirect effects of HIV may contribute to pathology, including proinflammatory cytokines and autoimmune mechanisms.[189] Cachexia and deficiencies of nutrients such as carnitine or selenium may play a role in certain settings. In advanced HIV disease, opportunistic and other infections can cause cardiac dysfunction, including but not limited to *Toxoplasma gondii*, *Pneumocystis jiroveci*, cytomegalovirus, Coxsackie virus, herpes simplex virus, cryptococcus, *Mycobacterium tuberculosis*, and *Mycobacterium avium complex*.[180,189,190] Mitochondrial toxicity from nucleoside reverse transcriptase inhibitors, including zidovudine and didanosine, likely can cause cardiomyopathy based on case reports and animal models.[191–193] Other drugs, such as pentamidine and anthracyclines, and illicit use of cocaine or methamphetamine may also contribute.

Diagnosis and Management

It is important to consider congestive heart failure due to dilated cardiomyopathy in the differential diagnosis of dyspnea in an HIV-infected patient. The differential diagnosis is broad and includes anemia, infectious etiologies (both routine and opportunistic pathogens), underlying pulmonary disease (e.g., chronic obstructive pulmonary disease [COPD], asthma), malignancy, and pulmonary hypertension (see Pulmonary Hypertension). The CD4 cell count, presence or absence of fever and other symptoms, physical examination (e.g., S3 gallop, rales, jugular venous distension, peripheral edema), and chest X-ray can narrow the differential diagnosis. Elevated plasma brain natriuretic peptide levels may be useful to support the diagnosis of congestive heart failure.[194]

Echocardiography is the principal diagnostic modality for cardiomyopathy but should not be done routinely as a screening test in the absence of symptoms and signs. Focal left ventricular dysfunction should prompt an evaluation for ischemic heart disease. An electrocardiogram (EKG) should also be done to assess for conduction abnormalities. Patients with CD4 cell counts <100 cell/mm^3 should have *Toxoplasma* serology and a serum cryptococcal antigen test. Acute and convalescent serologies for enteroviruses may be informative but are unlikely to affect clinical management. The role of endomyocardial biopsy in the evaluation of cardiomyopathy in HIV-infected patients is controversial and cannot be recommended routinely. Biopsy may be appropriate for patients with new-onset or rapid progression of symptoms,[195] lack of response to standard heart failure treatment,[196] or in the setting of positive *Toxoplasma* serology or serum cryptococcal antigenemia if the clinical suspicion of cardiac involvement is high.

Management of congestive heart failure/dilated cardiomyopathy does not differ in HIV-infected patients and includes diuretics, angiotensin-converting enzyme (ACE) inhibitors, and potentially β-blockers and digoxin. Patients on older NRTIs, such as zidovudine or didanosine, could be changed to other antiretrovirals based on treatment history and known resistance, although data on the efficacy of such switches are extremely limited and anecdotal.[192]

PRIMARY PULMONARY HYPERTENSION

Epidemiology

The prevalence of primary pulmonary hypertension in HIV-infected patients is approximately 0.5%, which is at least 10-fold and perhaps 100-fold more common than in the general population.[197] The available data suggest that the prevalence of pulmonary hypertension has not decreased in the current HIV treatment era relative to historical rates.[197,198]

Pathogenesis

The pathology of HIV-associated primary pulmonary hypertension is indistinguishable from idiopathic primary pulmonary hypertension. There is no evidence for direct infection of pulmonary endothelial cells, suggesting that HIV acts by indirect mechanisms, including the generation of growth factors and cytokines.[199] Other factors likely play a role in some patients, including genetic background[200] and illicit drug use, including cocaine and methamphetamine.[201]

Secondary causes of pulmonary hypertension include COPD, thromboembolic disease, sleep apnea, and left ventricular failure.[202] Of note, HIV-infected patients may be at increased risk of both accelerated emphysema[203] and venous thromboembolic disease.[204]

Diagnosis and Management

The clinical presentation of pulmonary hypertension is nonspecific, which may lead to delays in diagnosis. Patients may present with progressive dyspnea, nonproductive cough, fatigue, chest pain, and pedal edema. Physical examination may reveal a loud P2 (pulmonic part of the S2 heart sound) and signs of right ventricular failure. Although chest X-ray and EKG findings may be supportive, the key initial diagnostic test is echocardiogram with Doppler ultrasound. This technique uses the velocity of tricuspid regurgitation to estimate pulmonary artery pressure. Right heart catheterization is needed to confirm the diagnosis. Depending on the clinical suspicion for secondary causes, pulmonary function tests, high-resolution computed tomography (CT) of the chest, sleep studies, and ventilation/perfusion scanning may also be indicated.[202]

Ideally, patients with primary pulmonary hypertension should be managed at centers with expertise in this condition. Antiretroviral therapy should be initiated or optimized in patients who are viremic since limited, and conflicting, data suggest that antiretroviral therapy may improve pulmonary hypertension.[205,206] Small studies and case reports suggest that HIV-infected patients can be treated with standard drugs used to treat pulmonary hypertension, including bosentan,[207,208] epoprostenol,[209] sildenafil,[210] and calcium channel antagonists.[211] There is, however, potential for drug–drug interactions between PIs and both calcium channel antagonists[160] and sildenafil.[212,213] Supplemental oxygen and anticoagulation with warfarin are also cornerstones of therapy.[214]

PERICARDIAL DISEASE

Epidemiology

Studies completed before the highly active antiretroviral therapy (HAART) era documented pericardial effusion in about 20% of patients with AIDS.[180] The incidence of pericardial effusion was 11% per year in a longitudinal study employing serial echocardiogram in HIV-infected patients published in 1995.[215] Twelve of 13 patients who developed effusions had AIDS, and 80% had small, asymptomatic effusions. A small percentage of patients may present with pericarditis, large symptomatic effusions, or cardiac tamponade. The epidemiology of pericardial disease in the current HIV treatment era is not well characterized.

Pathogenesis

In most case series in the developed world, a substantial proportion of cases of pericardial disease are idiopathic,

Table 5 Causes of Pericardial Effusion in the HIV-Infected Patient[152]

Bacteria

- Staphylococcus aureus
- Streptococcus pneumoniae
- Enterococcus species
- Mycobacterium tuberculosis
- Mycobacterium avium complex
- Mycobacterium kansasii
- Nocardia asteroids
- Listeria monocytogenes
- Chlamydia trachomatis
- Proteus mirabilis
- Klebsiella pneumoniae
- Rhodococcus equi

Viruses

- Human immunodeficiency virus
- Herpes simplex virus
- Cytomegalovirus

Fungi

- Cryptococcus neoformans
- Histoplasma capsulatum
- Aspergillus species

Parasites

- Toxoplasma gondii

Malignancy

- Kaposi's sarcoma
- Non-Hodgkin's lymphoma
- Primary effusion lymphoma
- Adenocarcinoma

Other

- Idiopathic
- Hypothyroidism
- Wasting

whereas the remaining cases are due to infections or malignancy. Table 5 summarizes the potential causes of pericardial effusion in the HIV-infected patient.[180,216]

Diagnosis and Management

Asymptomatic pericardial effusions may be diagnosed incidentally by chest X-ray or echocardiogram done for other purposes. Patients with pericarditis may present with pleuritic chest pain with fever and may have a pericardial friction rub on physical examination. EKG findings in pericarditis include diffuse ST segment elevation, PR segment depression, and T-wave inversion. Patients with cardiac tamponade may have jugular venous distension, pulsus paradoxus, and sinus tachycardia. Echocardiogram is the diagnostic test of choice. There is no role for screening asymptomatic patients for pericardial effusion.

The major decision point in managing pericardial effusion is whether to observe the patient or to perform pericardiocentesis, typically by percutaneous catheter drainage, or surgical pericardiectomy. Most patients with small, asymptomatic pericardial effusions can be observed with periodic EKGs. Patients with cardiac tamponade, large effusions, or for whom there is clinical suspicion of malignant, purulent, or tuberculous effusion should undergo pericardiocentesis or pericardiectomy.[217,218] The diagnostic yield of pleural fluid examination varies and is typically reduced with chronic effusions (i.e., of >3 months' duration). In addition to routine biochemical analysis (glucose, protein, lactic dehydrogenase), cell counts, cytology, and microscopic stains and cultures, adenosine deaminase levels and polymerase chain reaction

(PCR) tests for *Mycobacterium tuberculosis* may help with diagnosis.[219] Additional diagnostic tests should include a purified protein derivative (PPD) test (although a negative test does not rule out tuberculous pericarditis) and potentially CT of the chest in stable patients to assess for tumor. Management depends on the specific diagnosis if one is made.

ENDOCARDITIS

Epidemiology

Limited data suggest that HIV-infected injection drug users with CD4 cell counts less than 350 cells/mm³ are at greater risk of infective endocarditis relative to HIV-uninfected injection drug users.[220] The spectrum of organisms causing endocarditis in HIV-infected patients is similar to that in the general population, where *Staphylococcus aureus* predominates.[221] The incidence of infective endocarditis may have decreased in the current HIV treatment era.[222] Management of infective endocarditis and the response to treatment do not differ in the HIV-infected patient, although advanced immunosuppression is associated with increased mortality.[223]

CARDIAC TUMORS

Cardiac involvement by AIDS-related malignancies is rare. Kaposi sarcoma of the heart is typically diagnosed postmortem and can involve the visceral layer of the serous pericardium and the subepicardial fat.[180] There are case reports of cardiac tamponade attributed to Kaposi sarcoma.[224,225] Disseminated non-Hodgkin lymphoma can involve the pericardium and/or myocardium.[226] Primary effusion lymphoma, which is caused by human herpesvirus-8 (also called Kaposi sarcoma–associated herpesvirus), can also affect the heart, manifesting as intracardiac mass, pericardial effusion, or potentially cardiac infiltration.[227,228]

CONDUCTION ABNORMALITIES

Cardiac conduction abnormalities are not infrequent in HIV-infected patients and can be related to the disease itself or to use of concomitant medications. The frequency of clinically significant abnormalities is not known. Prolongation of the QT interval can be seen in association with autonomic neuropathy in HIV-infected patients.[229] Several drugs used commonly in HIV-infected patients have also been associated with QT interval prolongation and torsades de pointes, including intravenous pentamidine and methadone.[230,231]

Although a theoretical basis exists for PIs to cause QT prolongation based on inhibition of ether-a-go-go-related gene (HERG) potassium channels *in vitro*,[232] in a large cross-sectional study, duration of HIV infection but not use of PIs was associated with QTc prolongation.[233] There are anecdotal reports of torsades de pointes in association with the use of the PI atazanavir, with or without concurrent methadone use[234,235] and the NNRTI efavirenz.[236] A recent update of the prescribing information for lopinavir/ritonavir notes that cases of QT interval prolongation and torsades de pointes have been reported with use of this drug, although causality is unknown.[237] Lopinavir/ritonavir should not be used in patients with congenital long QT syndrome, those with hypokalemia, and concurrently with other drugs that prolong the QT interval.[237]

PR interval prolongation has been reported in association with atazanavir use in a small prospective study of HIV-infected patients.[238] The prescribing information for atazanavir notes that PR interval prolongation and first-degree heart block have been seen in healthy volunteers and patients receiving the drug, and that there have been rare reports of second-degree heart block and other unspecified conduction abnormalities.[239] Atazanavir should be used with caution both in patients with preexisting conduction abnormalities and when concurrent use of drugs that prolong the PR interval is needed, especially drugs that are metabolized by cytochrome P450 3A4, such as verapamil or diltiazem.[239] Similarly, the prescribing information for lopinavir/ritonavir notes that PR interval prolongation and second- or third-degree heart block have been reported in association with its use.[237] Lopinavir/ritonavir should be used with caution in patients with underlying structural heart disease, preexisting conduction system abnormalities, ischemic heart disease, or cardiomyopathy, and when concurrent use of drugs that prolong the PR interval is needed, including calcium channel blockers, β-adrenergic blockers, and digoxin.[237]

Widening of the QRS interval and new asymptomatic bundle branch blocks have been reported in association with atazanavir use,[240] although the EKG methodology employed in that study has been questioned by scientists employed by the manufacturer of atazanavir.[241]

CLINICIAN RESOURCES

American Heart Association-American Academy of HIV Medicine: Initiative to Decrease Cardiovascular Risk and Increase Quality of Care for Patients Living with HIV/AIDS
http://www.americanheart.org/presenter.jhtml?identifier=3057579
AIDS Education and Training Centers:
Managing Dyslipidemia in HIV: A Comprehensive Tool for the Primary Care Clinician
http://www.aidsetc.org/aidsetc?page=etres-display&resource=etres-301
Management of Dyslipidemia in Adults Receiving Antiretroviral Therapy:
HIV Medicine Association of the Infectious Disease Society of America and the Adult AIDS Clinical Trials Group
http://www.idsociety.org/content.aspx?id=9202#md
Risk Assessment Tool for Estimating 10-year Risk of Developing Hard CHD (Myocardial Infarction and Coronary Death)
Framingham Risk Calculator
http://hp2010.nhlbihin.net/atpiii/calculator.asp?usertype=prof

PATIENT RESOURCES

Websites with information on cardiovascular disease in general and in the setting of HIV infection:
National Heart Lung and Blood Institute
http://www.nhlbi.nih.gov/chd/index.htm
Tufts University – HIV and Nutrition
http://www.tufts.edu/med/nutrition-infection/hiv/health_cvd.html
The Body: The Complete HIV/AIDS Resource
http://www.thebody.com/content/art50782.html
Gay Men's Health Crisis (GMHC) – Nutrition
http://www.gmhc.org/health/nutrition.html
AIDS Project Los Angeles
HIV Nutrition Fact Sheet: Lowering Cholesterol and Triglycerides
http://www.aidsetc.org/pdf/workgroups/pcare/Dyslipidemia_HIV_Nutrition_Education_Fact_Sheet.pdf

REFERENCES

1. Lohse N, Hansen AB, Pedersen G, et al. Survival of persons with and without HIV infection in Denmark, 1995–2005. *Ann Intern Med.* 2007;146:87–95.
2. Crum NF, Riffenburgh RH, Wegner S, et al. Comparisons of causes of death and mortality rates among HIV-infected persons: analysis of the pre-, early, and late HAART (highly active antiretroviral therapy) eras. *J Acquir Immune Defic Syndr.* 2006;41:194–200.
3. Palella FJ, Jr., Baker RK, Moorman AC, et al. Mortality in the highly active antir etroviral therapy era: changing causes of death and disease in the HIV outpatient study. *J Acquir Immune Defic Syndr.* 2006;43:27–34.
4. Sackoff JE, Hanna DB, Pfeiffer MR, et al. Causes of death among persons with AIDS in the era of highly active antiretroviral therapy: New York City. *Ann Intern Med.* 2006;145:397 406.
5. Henry K, Melroe H, Huebsch J, et al. Severe premature coronary artery disease with protease inhibitors. *Lancet.* 1998;351:1328.
6. Passalaris JD, Sepkowitz KA, Glesby MJ. Coronary artery disease and human immunodeficiency virus infection. *Clin Infect Dis.* 2000;31:787–797.
7. Currier JS, Taylor A, Boyd F, et al. Coronary heart disease in HIV-infected individuals. *J Acquir Immune Defic Syndr.* 2003;33:506–512.
8. Mary-Krause M, Cotte L, Simon A, et al. Increased risk of myocardial infarction with duration of protease inhibitor therapy in HIV-infected men. *AIDS.* 2003;17:2479–2486.
9. Obel N, Thomsen HF, Kronborg G, et al. Ischemic heart disease in HIV-infected and HIV-uninfected individuals: a population-based cohort study. *Clin Infect Dis.* 2007;44:1625–1631.
10. Triant VA, Lee H, Hadigan C, et al. Increased acute myocardial infarction rates and cardiovascular risk factors among patients with human immunodeficiency virus disease. *J Clin Endocrinol Metab.* 2007;92:2506–2512.
11. Klein D, Hurley LB, Quesenberry CPJ, et al. Do protease inhibitors increase the risk for coronary heart disease in patients with HIV-1 infection? *J Acquir Immune Defic Syndr.* 2002;30:471–477.

12. Friis-Moller N, Reiss P, Sabin CA, et al. Class of antiretroviral drugs and the risk of myocardial infarction. *N Engl J Med.* 2007;356:1723–1735.
13. Glass TR, Ungsedhapand C, Wolbers M, et al. Prevalence of risk factors for cardiovascular disease in HIV-infected patients over time: the Swiss HIV Cohort Study. *HIV Med.* 2006;7:404–410.
14. Sabin CA, d'Arminio MA, Friis-Moller N, et al. Changes over time in risk factors for cardiovascular disease and use of lipid-lowering drugs in HIV-infected individuals and impact on myocardial infarction. *Clin Infect Dis.* 2008;46:1101–1110.
15. Currier JS, Lundgren JD, Carr A, et al. Epidemiological evidence for cardiovascular disease in HIV-infected patients and relationship to highly active antiretroviral therapy. *Circulation.* 2008; 118:e29–e35.
16. Grunfeld C, Kotler DP, Hamadeh R, et al. Hypertriglyceridemia in the acquired immunodeficiency syndrome. *Am J Med.* 1989; 86:27–31.
17. Grunfeld C, Kotler DP, Shigenaga JK, et al. Circulating interferon-α levels and hypertriglyceridemia in the acquired immunodeficiency syndrome. *Am J Med.* 1991;90:154–162.
18. Feingold KR, Krauss RM, Pang M, et al. The hypertriglyceridemia of acquired immunodeficiency syndrome is associated with an increased prevalence of low density lipoprotein subclass pattern B. *J Clin Endocrinol Metab.* 1993;76:1423–1427.
19. Riddler SA, Smit E, Cole SR, et al. Impact of HIV infection and HAART on serum lipids in men. *JAMA.* 2003;289:2978–2982.
20. Shikuma CM, Yang Y, Glesby MJ, et al. Metabolic effects of protease inhibitor-sparing antiretroviral regimens given as initial treatment of HIV-1 Infection (AIDS Clinical Trials Group Study A5095). *J Acquir Immune Defic Syndr.* 2007;44:540–550.
21. Hammer SM, Eron JJ, Jr., Reiss P, et al. Antiretroviral treatment of adult HIV infection: 2008 recommendations of the International AIDS Society-USA panel. *JAMA.* 2008;300: 555–570.
22. Panel on Antiretroviral Guidelines for Adult and Adolescents. Guidelines for the use of antiretroviral agents in HIV-1–infected adults and adolescents. 2008. Department of Health and Human

Services. November 3, 2008;1–139. Available at: http://www.aidsinfo.nih.gov/ContentFiles/AdultandAdolescentGL.pdf. Accessed August 14, 2009.

23. Lennox JL, DeJesus E, Lazzarin A, et al. Safety and efficacy of raltegravir-based versus efavirenz-based combination therapy in treatment-naive patients with HIV-1 infection: a multicentre, double-blind randomised controlled trial. *Lancet*. 2009.

24. Gallant JE, Staszewski S, Pozniak AL, et al. Efficacy and safety of tenofovir DF vs stavudine in combination therapy in antiretroviral-naive patients: a 3-year randomized trial. *JAMA*. 2004;292:191–201.

25. Tungsiripat M, Kitch D, Glesby M, et al. A pilot study to determine the effect on dyslipidemia of the addition of tenofovir to stable background ART in HIV-infected subjects: results from the A5206 Study Team [abstr 714]. Program and Abstracts of the 16th Conference on Retroviruses and Opportunistic Infections, Montreal, PQ, Feb 8–11, 2009. 2009.

26. Anastos K, Lu D, Shi Q, et al. Association of serum lipid levels with HIV serostatus, specific antiretroviral agents, and treatment regimens. *J Acquir Immune Defic Syndr*. 2007;45:34–42.

27. Moyle GJ, Baldwin C, Langroudi B, et al. A 48-week, randomized, open-label comparison of three abacavir-based substitution approaches in the management of dyslipidemia and peripheral lipoatrophy. *J Acquir Immune Defic Syndr*. 2003;33:22–28.

28. Keiser PH, Sension MG, DeJesus E, et al. Substituting abacavir for hyperlipidemia-associated protease inhibitors in HAART regimens improves fasting lipid profiles, maintains virologic suppression, and simplifies treatment. *BMC Infect Dis*. 2005;5:2.

29. van Leth F, Phanuphak P, Stroes E, et al. Nevirapine and Efavirenz Elicit Different Changes in Lipid Profiles in Antiretroviral- Therapy-Naive Patients Infected with HIV-1. *Plos Med*. 2004;1:e19.

30. Roberts AD, Liappis AP, Chinn C, et al. Effect of delavirdine on plasma lipids and lipoproteins in patients receiving antiretroviral therapy. *AIDS*. 2002;16:1829–1830.

31. Campbell T, Grinsztejn B, Hartikainen J, et al. Long-term safety profile of etravirine in treatment-experienced, HIV-1–

infected patients: pooled 96-week results from the phase III DUET trials [abstr MOPEB038]. Program and Abstracts of the 5th IAS Conference on HIV Pathogenesis, Treatment and Prevention, Cape Town, South Africa, July 19–22, 2009.

32. Malan DR, Krantz E, David N, et al. Efficacy and safety of atazanavir, with or without ritonavir, as part of once-daily highly active antiretroviral therapy regimens in antiretroviral-naive patients. *J Acquir Immune Defic Syndr.* 2008;47:161–167.

33. Rodriguez-French A, Boghossian J, Gray GE, et al. The NEAT study: a 48-week open-label study to compare the antiviral efficacy and safety of GW433908 versus nelfinavir in antiretroviral therapy-naive HIV-1–infected patients. *J Acquir Immune Defic Syndr.* 2004;35:22–32.

34. Eron J, Jr., Yeni P, Gathe J, Jr., et al. The KLEAN study of fosamprenavir-ritonavir versus lopinavir-ritonavir, each in combination with abacavir-lamivudine, for initial treatment of HIV infection over 48 weeks: a randomised non-inferiority trial. *Lancet.* 2006;368:476–482.

35. Smith KY, Weinberg WG, DeJesus E, et al. Fosamprenavir or atazanavir once daily boosted with ritonavir 100 mg, plus tenofovir/emtricitabine, for the initial treatment of HIV infection: 48-week results of ALERT. *AIDS Res Ther.* 2008;5:5.

36. Smith KY, Patel P, Fine D, et al. Randomized, double-blind, placebo-matched, multicenter trial of abacavir/lamivudine or tenofovir/emtricitabine with lopinavir/ritonavir for initial HIV treatment. *AIDS.* 2009;23:1547–1556.

37. Saag M, Ive P, Heere J, et al. A multicenter, randomized, double-blind, comparative trial of a novel CCR5 antagonist, maraviroc vs efavirenz, both in combination with combivir (zidovudine/lamivudine), for the treatment of antiretroviral naive patients infected with R5 HIV-1: week 48 results of the MERIT study [abstr WESS104]. Program and Abstracts of the 4th IAS Conference on HIV Pathogenesis, Treatment and Prevention, Sydney, Australia, July 22–25, 2007.

38. Markowitz M, Nguyen BY, Gotuzzo E, et al. Rapid and durable antiretroviral effect of the HIV-1 Integrase inhibitor raltegravir as part of combination therapy in treatment-naive

patients with HIV-1 infection: results of a 48-week controlled study. *J Acquir Immune Defic Syndr.* 2007;46:125–133.
39. Lalezari JP, Henry K, O'Hearn M, et al. Enfuvirtide, an HIV-1 fusion inhibitor, for drug-resistant HIV infection in North and South America. *N Engl J Med.* 2003;348:2175–2185.
40. Sabin CA, Worm SW, Weber R, et al. Use of nucleoside reverse transcriptase inhibitors and risk of myocardial infarction in HIV-infected patients enrolled in the D:A:D study: a multi-cohort collaboration. *Lancet.* 2008;371:1417–1426.
41. The SMART/INSIGHT and the D:A:D Study Groups. Use of nucleoside reverse transcriptase inhibitors and risk of myocardial infarction in HIV-infected patients. AIDS 22, F17–F24. 2008.
42. Benson C, Ribaudo H, Zheng E, et al., and the ACTG A5001/ALLRT Protocol Team. No association of abacavir use with risk of myocardial infarction or severe cardiovascular disease events: results from ACTG A5001 [abstr 721]. Program and Abstracts of the 16th Conference on Retroviruses and Opportunistic Infections, Montreal, PQ, Feb 8–11, 2009. 2009.
43. Brothers CH, Hernandez JE, Cutrell AG, et al. Risk of myocardial infarction and abacavir therapy: no increased risk across 52 GlaxoSmithKline-sponsored clinical trials in adult subjects. *J Acquir Immune Defic Syndr.* 2009;51:20–28.
44. Bedimo R, Westfall A, Drechsler H, Tebas P. Abacavir use and risk of acute myocardial infarction and cerebrovascular disease in the HAART era [abstr MOAB202]. Program and Abstracts of the 5th IAS Conference on HIV Pathogenesis, Treatment and Prevention, Cape Town, South Africa, July 19–22, 2009.
45. Pereg D, Tirosh A, Shochat T, et al. Mild renal dysfunction associated with incident coronary artery disease in young males. *Eur Heart J.* 2008;29:198–203.
46. Van Biesen W, De Bacquer D, Verbeke F, et al. The glomerular filtration rate in an apparently healthy population and its relation with cardiovascular mortality during 10 years. *Eur Heart J.* 2007;28:478–483.
47. Hallan S, Astor B, Romundstad S, et al. Association of kidney function and albuminuria with cardiovascular mortality in older vs younger individuals: The HUNT II Study. *Arch Intern Med.* 2007;167:2490–2496.

48. Hsue PY, Hunt PW, Wu Y, et al. Association of abacavir and impaired endothelial function in treated and suppressed HIV-infected patients. *AIDS*. 2009.
49. Hammond E, McKinnon E, Mallal S, et al. Longitudinal evaluation of cardiovascular disease-associated biomarkers in relation to abacavir therapy. *AIDS*. 2008;22:2540–2543.
50. El Sadr WM, Lundgren JD, Neaton JD, et al. CD4+ count-guided interruption of antiretroviral treatment. *N Engl J Med*. 2006;355:2283–2296.
51. Phillips AN, Carr A, Neuhaus J, et al. Interruption of antiretroviral therapy and risk of cardiovascular disease in persons with HIV-1 infection: exploratory analyses from the SMART trial. *Antivir Ther*. 2008;13:177–187.
52. Kuller LH, Tracy R, Belloso W, et al. Inflammatory and coagulation biomarkers and mortality in patients with HIV infection. *Plos Med*. 2008;5:e203.
53. Hsue PY, Hunt PW, Schnell A, et al. Role of viral replication, antiretroviral therapy, and immunodeficiency in HIV-associated atherosclerosis. *AIDS*. 2009;23:1059–1067.
54. Henry K, Kitch D, Dube M, et al. C-Reactive protein levels over time and cardiovascular risk in HIV-infected individuals suppressed on an indinavir-based regimen: AIDS Clinical Trials Group 5056s. *AIDS*. 2004;18:2434–2437.
55. Shikuma C, Zheng E, Ribaudo H, et al., and AIDS Clinical Trials Group A5095. 96-week effects of suppressive efavirenz-containing ART, abacavir, and sex on high-sensitivity C-reactive protein: ACTG A5095 [abstr 736]. Program and Abstracts of the 16th Conference on Retroviruses and Opportunistic Infections, Montreal, PQ, Feb 8–11, 2009.
56. Triant VA, Meigs JB, Grinspoon SK. Association of C-reactive protein and HIV infection with acute myocardial infarction. *J Acquir Immune Defic Syndr*. 2009;51:268–273.
57. Hsue PY, Hunt PW, Sinclair E, et al. Increased carotid intima-media thickness in HIV patients is associated with increased cytomegalovirus-specific T-cell responses. *AIDS*. 2006;20:2275–2283.
58. Freiberg MS, Cheng DM, Kraemer KL, et al. The association between hepatitis C infection and prevalent cardiovascular disease among HIV-infected individuals. *AIDS*. 2007;21:193–197.

59. Tien PC, Schneider MF, Cole SR, et al. Association of hepatitis C virus and HIV infection with subclinical atherosclerosis in the women's interagency HIV study. *AIDS*. 2009.
60. Brown TT, Cole SR, Li X, et al. Antiretroviral therapy and the prevalence and incidence of diabetes mellitus in the multicenter AIDS cohort study. *Arch Intern Med*. 2005;165:1179–1184.
61. Butt AA, McGinnis K, Rodriguez-Barradas MC, et al. HIV infection and the risk of diabetes mellitus. *AIDS*. 2009;23:1227–1234.
62. Dube MP. Disorders of glucose metabolism in patients infected with human immunodeficiency virus. *Clin Infect Dis*. 2000;31:1467–1475.
63. Tien PC, Schneider MF, Cole SR, et al. Antiretroviral therapy exposure and incidence of diabetes mellitus in the Women's Interagency HIV Study. *AIDS*. 2007;21:1739–1745.
64. Tien PC, Schneider MF, Cole SR, et al. Antiretroviral therapy exposure and insulin resistance in the Women's Interagency HIV study. *J Acquir Immune Defic Syndr*. 2008;49:369–376.
65. Fleischman A, Johnsen S, Systrom DM, et al. Effects of a nucleoside reverse transcriptase inhibitor, stavudine, on glucose disposal and mitochondrial function in muscle of healthy adults. *Am J Physiol Endocrinol Metab*. 2007;292:E1666–E1673.
66. De Wit S, Sabin CA, Weber R, et al. Incidence and risk factors for new-onset diabetes in HIV-infected patients: the Data Collection on Adverse Events of Anti-HIV Drugs (D:A:D) study. *Diabetes Care*. 2008;31:1224–1229.
67. Noor MA, Seneviratne T, Aweeka FT, et al. Indinavir acutely inhibits insulin-stimulated glucose disposal in humans: a randomized, placebo-controlled study. *AIDS*. 2002;16:F1–F8.
68. Murata H, Hruz PW, Mueckler M. The mechanism of insulin resistance caused by HIV protease inhibitor therapy. *J Biol Chem*. 2000;275:20251–20254.
69. Carr A, Samaras K, Burton S, et al. A syndrome of peripheral lipodystrophy, hyperlipidaemia and insulin resistance in patients receiving HIV protease inhibitors. *Lancet*. 1998;12:F51–F58.
70. Martinez E, Mocroft A, Garcia-Viejo MA, et al. Risk of lipodystrophy in HIV-1–infected patients treated with protease inhibitors: a prospective cohort study. *Lancet*. 2001;357:592–598.

71. Miller KK, Daly PA, Sentochnik D, et al. Pseudo-Cushing's syndrome in human immunodeficiency virus-infected patients. *Clin Infect Dis.* 1998;27:68–72.

72. Bacchetti P, Gripshover B, Grunfeld C, et al. Fat distribution in men with HIV infection. *J Acquir Immune Defic Syndr.* 2005;40:121–131.

73. Study of Fat Redistribution and Metabolic Change in HIV Infection (FRAM). Fat distribution in women with HIV infection. *J Acquir Immune Defic Syndr.* 2006;42:562–571.

74. Tien PC, Cole SR, Williams CM, et al. Incidence of lipoatrophy and lipohypertrophy in the women's interagency HIV study. *J Acquir Immune Defic Syndr.* 2003;34:461–466.

75. Hadigan C, Meigs JB, Corcoran C, et al. Metabolic abnormalities and cardiovascular disease risk factors in adults with human immunodeficiency virus infection and lipodystrophy. *Clin Infect Dis.* 2001;32:130–139.

76. Mynarcik DC, McNurlan MA, Steigbigel RT, et al. Association of severe insulin resistance with both loss of limb fat and elevated serum tumor necrosis factor receptor levels in HIV lipodystrophy. *J Acquir Immune Defic Syndr.* 2000;25:312–321.

77. Balasubramanyam A, Sekhar RV, Jahoor F, et al. Pathophysiology of dyslipidemia and increased cardiovascular risk in HIV lipodystrophy: a model of 'systemic steatosis'. *Curr Opin Lipidol.* 2004;15:59–67.

78. Dubé MP, Komarow L, Mulligan K, Grinspoon SK, Parker RA, Robbins GK, Roubenoff R, Tebas P; Adult Clinical Trials Group 384. Long-term body fat outcomes in antiretroviral-naive participants randomized to nelfinavir or efavirenz or both plus dual nucleosides. Dual X-ray absorptiometry results from A5005s, a substudy of Adult Clinical Trials Group 384. *J Acquir Immune Defic Syndr.* 2007 Aug 15;45(5):508–14.

79. Lichtenstein KA, Ward DJ, Moorman AC, et al. Clinical assessment of HIV-associated lipodystrophy in an ambulatory population. *AIDS.* 2001;15:1389–1398.

80. Joly V, Flandre P, Meiffredy V, et al. Increased risk of lipoatrophy under stavudine in HIV-1–infected patients: results of a substudy from a comparative trial. *AIDS.* 2002;16:2447–2454.

81. McComsey GA, Paulsen DM, Lonergan JT, et al. Improvements in lipoatrophy, mitochondrial DNA levels and fat apoptosis after replacing stavudine with abacavir or zidovudine. *AIDS*. 2005;19:15–23.
82. Baekken M, Os I, Sandvik L, et al. Hypertension in an urban HIV-positive population compared with the general population: influence of combination antiretroviral therapy. *J Hypertens*. 2008;26:2126–2133.
83. Khalsa A, Karim R, Mack WJ, et al. Correlates of prevalent hypertension in a large cohort of HIV-infected women: Women's Interagency HIV Study. *AIDS*. 2007;21:2539–2541.
84. Palacios R, Santos J, Garcia A, et al. Impact of highly active antiretroviral therapy on blood pressure in HIV-infected patients. A prospective study in a cohort of naive patients. *HIV Med*. 2006;7:10–15.
85. Grandominico JM, Fichtenbaum CJ. Short term effect of HAART on blood pressure in HIV-infected individuals. *HIV Clin Trials*. 2008;9:52–60.
86. Seaberg EC, Munoz A, Lu M, et al. Association between highly active antiretroviral therapy and hypertension in a large cohort of men followed from 1984 to 2003. *AIDS*. 2005;19:953–960.
87. Thiebaut R, El Sadr WM, Friis-Moller N, et al. Predictors of hypertension and changes of blood pressure in HIV-infected patients. *Antivir Ther*. 2005;10:811–823.
88. Cattelan AM, Trevenzoli M, Sasset L, et al. Indinavir and systemic hypertension. *AIDS*. 2001;15:805–807.
89. Cattelan AM, Trevenzoli M, Naso A, et al. Severe hypertension and renal atrophy associated with indinavir. *Clin Infect Dis*. 2000;30:619–621.
90. Sattler FR, Qian D, Louie S, et al. Elevated blood pressure in subjects with lipodystrophy. *AIDS*. 2001;15:2001–2010.
91. Crane HM, Grunfeld C, Harrington RD, et al. Lipoatrophy and lipohypertrophy are independently associated with hypertension. *HIV Med*. 2009.
92. Kimmel PL, Barisoni L, Kopp JB. Pathogenesis and treatment of HIV-associated renal diseases: lessons from clinical and

animal studies, molecular pathologic correlations, and genetic investigations. *Ann Intern Med.* 2003;139:214–226.
93. Winston J, Deray G, Hawkins T, et al. Kidney disease in patients with HIV infection and AIDS. *Clin Infect Dis.* 2008;47:1449–1457.
94. Torriani FJ, Komarow L, Parker RA, et al. Endothelial function in human immunodeficiency virus-infected antiretroviral-naive subjects before and after starting potent antiretroviral therapy: The ACTG (AIDS Clinical Trials Group) Study 5152s. *J Am Coll Cardiol.* 2008;52:569–576.
95. Stein JH, Klein MA, Bellehumeur JL, et al. Use of human immunodeficiency virus-1 protease inhibitors is associated with atherogenic lipoprotein changes and endothelial dysfunction. *Circulation.* 2001;104:257–262.
96. Dube MP, Gorski JC, Shen C. Severe impairment of endothelial function with the HIV-1 protease inhibitor indinavir is not mediated by insulin resistance in healthy subjects. *Cardiovasc Toxicol.* 2008;8:15–22.
97. Mondy KE, de las FL, Waggoner A, et al. Insulin resistance predicts endothelial dysfunction and cardiovascular risk in HIV-infected persons on long-term highly active antiretroviral therapy. *AIDS.* 2008;22:849–856.
98. Sabin CA, Worm SW. Conventional cardiovascular risk factors in HIV infection: how conventional are they? *Curr Opin HIV AIDS.* 2008;3:214–219.
99. Amorosa V, Synnestvedt M, Gross R, et al. A tale of 2 epidemics: the intersection between obesity and HIV infection in Philadelphia. *J Acquir Immune Defic Syndr.* 2005;39:557–561.
100. Qureshi AI, Suri MF, Guterman LR, et al. Cocaine use and the likelihood of nonfatal myocardial infarction and stroke: data from the Third National Health and Nutrition Examination Survey. *Circulation.* 2001;103:502–506.
101. Yu Q, Larson DF, Watson RR. Heart disease, methamphetamine and AIDS. *Life Sci.* 2003;73:129–140.
102. Lai S, Lai H, Meng Q, et al. Effect of cocaine use on coronary calcium among black adults in Baltimore, Maryland. *Am J Cardiol.* 2002;90:326–328.

103. Dube MP, Stein JH, Aberg JA, et al. Guidelines for the evaluation and management of dyslipidemia in human immunodeficiency virus (HIV)-infected adults receiving antiretroviral therapy: recommendations of the HIV Medical Association of the Infectious Disease Society of America and the Adult AIDS Clinical Trials Group. *Clin Infect Dis.* 2003;37:613–627.

104. Schambelan M, Benson CA, Carr A, et al. Management of metabolic complications associated with antiretroviral therapy for HIV-1 infection: recommendations of an International AIDS Society-USA panel. *J Acquir Immune Defic Syndr.* 2002;31:257–275.

105. Evans SR, Fichtenbaum CJ, Aberg JA. Comparison of direct and indirect measurement of LDL-C in HIV-infected individuals: ACTG 5087. *HIV Clin Trials.* 2007;8:45–52.

106. Baigent C, Blackwell L, Collins R, et al. Aspirin in the primary and secondary prevention of vascular disease: collaborative meta-analysis of individual participant data from randomised trials. *Lancet.* 2009;373:1849–1860.

107. Wolff T, Miller T, Ko S. Aspirin for the primary prevention of cardiovascular events: an update of the evidence for the U.S. Preventive Services Task Force. *Ann Intern Med.* 2009;150:405–410.

108. Elzi L, Spoerl D, Voggensperger J, et al. A smoking cessation programme in HIV-infected individuals: a pilot study. *Antivir Ther.* 2006;11:787–795.

109. Tashima K, Niaura R, Richardson E, et al. Positive Paths: a motivational intervention for smoking cessation among HIV+ smokers [abstr 148]. Program and Abstracts of the 16th Conference on Retroviruses and Opportunistic Infections, Montreal, PQ, Feb 8–11, 2009. 2009.

110. Hesse LM, Greenblatt DJ, von Moltke LL, et al. Ritonavir has minimal impact on the pharmacokinetic disposition of a single dose of bupropion administered to human volunteers. *J Clin Pharmacol.* 2006;46:567–576.

111. Hogeland GW, Swindells S, McNabb JC, et al. Lopinavir/ritonavir reduces bupropion plasma concentrations in healthy subjects. *Clin Pharmacol Ther.* 2007;81:69–75.

112. Anonymous. The smoking cessation aids varenicline (marketed as Chantix) and bupropion (marketed as Zyban and generics): suicidal ideation and behavior. FDA Drug Safety Newsletter, Vol. 2, No 1, 2009. Available at: http://www.fda.gov/downloads/Drugs/DrugSafety/DrugSafetyNewsletter/ucm107318.pdf. Accessed 8/14/09.

113. Executive Summary of The Third Report of The National Cholesterol Education Program (NCEP) Expert Panel on Detection, Evaluation, And Treatment of High Blood Cholesterol In Adults (Adult Treatment Panel III). *JAMA*. 2001;285:2486–2497.

114. Law MG, Friis-Moller N, El Sadr WM, et al. The use of the Framingham equation to predict myocardial infarctions in HIV-infected patients: comparison with observed events in the D:A:D Study. *HIV Med*. 2006;7:218–230.

115. Bernal E, Masia M, Padilla S, et al. High-density lipoprotein cholesterol in HIV-infected patients: evidence for an association with HIV-1 viral load, antiretroviral therapy status, and regimen composition. *AIDS Patient Care STDS*. 2008;22:569–575.

116. Pate RR, Pratt M, Blair SN, et al. Physical activity and public health. A recommendation from the Centers for Disease Control and Prevention and the American College of Sports Medicine. *JAMA*. 1995;273:402–407.

117. Joy T, Keogh HM, Hadigan C, et al. Dietary fat intake and relationship to serum lipid levels in HIV-infected patients with metabolic abnormalities in the HAART era. *AIDS*. 2007;21:1591–1600.

118. National Cholesterol Education Program (NCEP) Expert Panel on Detection EaToHBCiAATPI. Third Report of the National Cholesterol Education Program (NCEP) Expert Panel on Detection, Evaluation, and Treatment of High Blood Cholesterol in Adults (Adult Treatment Panel III) final report. Circulation 106, 3143–3421. 2002.

119. Barrios A, Blanco F, Garcia-Benayas T, et al. Effect of dietary intervention on highly active antiretroviral therapy-related dyslipidemia. *AIDS*. 2002;16:2079–2081.

120. Jones SP, Doran DA, Leatt PB, et al. Short-term exercise training improves body composition and hyperlipidaemia in HIV-positive individuals with lipodystrophy. *AIDS*. 2001;15:2049–2051.

121. Calza L, Manfredi R, Colangeli V, et al. Substitution of nevirapine or efavirenz for protease inhibitor versus lipid-lowering therapy for the management of dyslipidaemia. *AIDS*. 2005;19:1051–1058.

122. Fisac C, Fumero E, Crespo M, et al. Metabolic benefits 24 months after replacing a protease inhibitor with abacavir, efavirenz or nevirapine. *AIDS*. 2005;19:917–925.

123. Gatell J, Salmon-Ceron D, Lazzarin A, et al. Efficacy and safety of atazanavir-based highly active antiretroviral therapy in patients with virologic suppression switched from a stable, boosted or unboosted protease inhibitor treatment regimen: the SWAN Study (AI424–097) 48-week results. *Clin Infect Dis*. 2007;44:1484–1492.

124. Sension M, Andrade Neto JL, Grinsztejn B, et al. Improvement in lipid profiles in antiretroviral-experienced HIV-positive patients with hyperlipidemia after a switch to unboosted atazanavir. *J Acquir Immune Defic Syndr*. 2009;51:153–162.

125. Moyle GJ, Sabin CA, Cartledge J, et al. A randomized comparative trial of tenofovir DF or abacavir as replacement for a thymidine analogue in persons with lipoatrophy. *AIDS*. 2006;20:2043–2050.

126. Eron J, Andrade J, Rajdenverg R, et al. Switching from stable lopinavir/ritonavir-based to raltegravir-based combination art resulted in a superior lipid profile at week 12 but did not demonstrate non-inferior virologic efficacy at week 24 [abstr 70aLB]. Program and Abstracts of the 16th Conference on Retroviruses and Opportunistic Infections, Montreal, PQ, Feb 8–11, 2009.

127. Eckhardt BJ, Glesby MJ. Antiretroviral therapy and cardiovascular risk: are some medications cardioprotective? *Curr Opin HIV AIDS*. 2008;3:226–233.

128. Fichtenbaum CJ, Gerber JG, Rosenkranz SL, et al. Pharmacokinetic interactions between protease inhibitors and statins in HIV seronegative volunteers: ACTG Study A5047. *AIDS*. 2002;16:569–577.

129. Aberg JA, Rosenkranz SL, Fichtenbaum CJ, et al. Pharmacokinetic interaction between nelfinavir and pravastatin in HIV-seronegative volunteers: ACTG Study A5108. *AIDS*. 2006;20:725–729.

130. Sekar VJ, Spinosa-Guzman S, Marien K,, et al. Pharmacokinetic drug-drug interaction between the new HIV protease inhibitor darunavir (TMC114) and the lipid-lowering agent pravastatin [abstr 55]. Program and Abstracts of the 8th International Workshop on Pharmacology of HIV Therapy, Budapest, Hungary, April 16–18, 2007. 2007.

131. Kiser JJ, Gerber JG, Predhomme JA, et al. Drug/Drug interaction between lopinavir/ritonavir and rosuvastatin in healthy volunteers. *J Acquir Immune Defic Syndr*. 2008;47:570–578.

132. Hare CB, Vu MP, Grunfeld C, et al. Simvastatin-nelfinavir interaction implicated in rhabdomyolysis and death. *Clin Infect Dis*. 2002;35:e111–e112.

133. Moyle GJ, Lloyd M, Reynolds B, et al. Dietary advice with or without pravastatin for the management of hypercholesterolaemia associated with protease inhibitor therapy. *AIDS*. 2001;15:1503–1508.

134. Aberg JA, Zackin RA, Brobst SW, et al. A randomized trial of the efficacy and safety of fenofibrate versus pravastatin in HIV-infected subjects with lipid abnormalities: AIDS Clinical Trials Group Study 5087. *AIDS Res Hum Retroviruses*. 2005;21:757–767.

135. Darunavir (Prezista) prescribing information. 2009. Raritan, NJ, Tibotec, Inc., June 2009 (package insert).

136. Gerber JG, Rosenkranz SL, Fichtenbaum CJ, et al. Effect of efavirenz on the pharmacokinetics of simvastatin, atorvastatin, and pravastatin: results of AIDS clinical trials group 5108 study. *J Acquir Immune Defic Syndr*. 2005;39:307–312.

137. Miller J, Brown D, Amin J, et al. A randomized, double-blind study of gemfibrozil for the treatment of protease inhibitor-associated hypertriglyceridaemia. *AIDS*. 2002;16:2195–2200.

138. Gerber MT, Mondy KE, Yarasheski KE, et al. Niacin in HIV-infected individuals with hyperlipidemia receiving potent antiretroviral therapy. *Clin Infect Dis*. 2004;39:419–425.

139. Dube MP, Wu JW, Aberg JA, et al. Safety and efficacy of extended-release niacin for the treatment of dyslipidaemia in patients with HIV infection: AIDS Clinical Trials Group Study A5148. *Antivir Ther.* 2006;11:1081–1089.

140. Wohl DA, Tien HC, Busby M, et al. Randomized study of the safety and efficacy of fish oil (omega-3 fatty acid) supplementation with dietary and exercise counseling for the treatment of antiretroviral therapy-associated hypertriglyceridemia. *Clin Infect Dis.* 2005;41:1498–1504.

141. Gerber JG, Kitch DW, Fichtenbaum CJ, et al. Fish oil and fenofibrate for the treatment of hypertriglyceridemia in HIV-infected subjects on antiretroviral therapy: results of ACTG A5186. *J Acquir Immune Defic Syndr.* 2008;47:459–466.

142. de Truchis P, Kirstetter M, Perier A, et al. Reduction in triglyceride level with N-3 polyunsaturated fatty acids in HIV-infected patients taking potent antiretroviral therapy: a randomized prospective study. *J Acquir Immune Defic Syndr.* 2007;44:278–285.

143. Rosenson RS. Current overview of statin-induced myopathy. *Am J Med.* 2004;116:408–416.

144. Chow DC, Chen H, Glesby MJ, et al. Short term ezetimibe is well tolerated and effective in combination with statin therapy to treat elevated LDL cholesterol in HIV-infected participants: ACTG 5209. In press, *AIDS.* 2009.

145. Kastelein JJ, Akdim F, Stroes ES, et al. Simvastatin with or without ezetimibe in familial hypercholesterolemia. *N Engl J Med.* 2008;358:1431–1443.

146. Rossebo AB, Pedersen TR, Boman K, et al. Intensive lipid lowering with simvastatin and ezetimibe in aortic stenosis. *N Engl J Med.* 2008;359:1343–1356.

147. Peto R, Emberson J, Landray M, et al. Analyses of cancer data from three ezetimibe trials. *N Engl J Med.* 2008;359:1357–1366.

148. Kohli R, Shevitz A, Gorbach S, et al. A randomized placebo-controlled trial of metformin for the treatment of HIV lipodystrophy. *HIV Med.* 2007;8:420–426.

149. Hadigan C, Corcoran C, Basgoz N, et al. Metformin in the treatment of HIV lipodystrophy syndrome: A randomized controlled trial. *JAMA.* 2000;284:472–477.

150. Mulligan K, Yang Y, Wininger DA, et al. Effects of metformin and rosiglitazone in HIV-infected patients with hyperinsulinemia and elevated waist/hip ratio. *AIDS*. 2007;21:47–57.
151. van Wijk JP, de Koning EJ, Cabezas MC, et al. Comparison of rosiglitazone and metformin for treating HIV lipodystrophy: a randomized trial. *Ann Intern Med*. 2005;143:337–346.
152. Lonergan JT, McComsey GA, Fisher RL, et al. Lack of recurrence of hyperlactatemia in HIV-infected patients switched from stavudine to abacavir or zidovudine. *J Acquir Immune Defic Syndr*. 2004;36:935–942.
153. Lonergan JT, Barber RE, Mathews WC. Safety and efficacy of switching to alternative nucleoside analogues following symptomatic hyperlactatemia and lactic acidosis. *AIDS*. 2003;17:2495–2499.
154. Hocqueloux L, Alberti C, Feugeas JP, et al. Prevalence, risk factors and outcome of hyperlactataemia in HIV-infected patients. *HIV Med*. 2003;4:18–23.
155. Kim PS, Woods C, Georgoff P, et al. Hemoglobin A1c Underestimates Glycemia in HIV Infection. *Diabetes Care*. 2009.
156. Armbruster DA. Fructosamine: structure, analysis, and clinical usefulness. *Clin Chem*. 1987;33:2153–2163.
157. Samaras K. Prevalence and pathogenesis of diabetes mellitus in HIV-1 infection treated with combined antiretroviral therapy. *J Acquir Immune Defic Syndr*. 2009;50:499–505.
158. Nathan DM, Davidson MB, DeFronzo RA, et al. Impaired fasting glucose and impaired glucose tolerance: implications for care. *Diabetes Care*. 2007;30:753–759.
159. Salpeter SR, Buckley NS, Kahn JA, et al. Meta-analysis: metformin treatment in persons at risk for diabetes mellitus. *Am J Med*. 2008;121:149–157.
160. Glesby MJ, Aberg JA, Kendall MA, et al. Pharmacokinetic interactions between indinavir plus ritonavir and calcium channel blockers. *Clin Pharmacol Ther*. 2005;78:143–153.
161. Fichtenbaum CJ, Gerber JG. Interactions between antiretroviral drugs and drugs used for the therapy of the metabolic complications encountered during HIV infection. *Clin Pharmacokinet*. 2002;41:1195–1211.

162. Folsom AR, Kushi LH, Anderson KE, et al. Associations of general and abdominal obesity with multiple health outcomes in older women: the Iowa Women's Health Study. *Arch Intern Med.* 2000;160:2117–2128.
163. Yusuf S, Hawken S, Ounpuu S, et al. Effect of potentially modifiable risk factors associated with myocardial infarction in 52 countries (the INTERHEART study): case-control study. *Lancet.* 2004;364:937–952.
164. Grunfeld C, Thompson M, Brown SJ, et al. Recombinant human growth hormone to treat HIV-associated adipose redistribution syndrome: 12 week induction and 24-week maintenance therapy. *J Acquir Immune Defic Syndr.* 2007;45:286–297.
165. Falutz J, Allas S, Blot K, et al. Metabolic effects of a growth hormone-releasing factor in patients with HIV. *N Engl J Med.* 2007;357:2359–2370.
166. Thoni GJ, Fedou C, Brun JF, et al. Reduction of fat accumulation and lipid disorders by individualized light aerobic training in human immunodeficiency virus infected patients with lipodystrophy and/or dyslipidemia. *Diabetes Metab.* 2002;28:397–404.
167. Roubenoff R, Schmitz H, Bairos L, et al. Reduction of abdominal obesity in lipodystrophy associated with human immunodeficiency virus infection by means of diet and exercise: case report and proof of principle. *Clin Infect Dis.* 2002;34:390–393.
168. Hansen BR, Haugaard SB, Iversen J, et al. Impact of switching antiretroviral therapy on lipodystrophy and other metabolic complications: a review. *Scand J Infect Dis.* 2004;36:244–253.
169. Hadigan C, Meigs JB, Rabe J, et al. Increased PAI-1 and tPA antigen levels are reduced with metformin therapy in HIV-infected patients with fat redistribution and insulin resistance. *J Clin Endocrinol Metab.* 2001;86:939–943.
170. Driscoll SD, Meininger GE, Lareau MT, et al. Effects of exercise training and metformin on body composition and cardiovascular indices in HIV-infected patients. *AIDS.* 2004;18:465–473.
171. Carr A, Workman C, Smith DE, et al. Abacavir substitution for nucleoside analogs in patients with HIV lipoatrophy: a randomized trial. *JAMA.* 2002;288:207–215.

172. Martin A, Smith DE, Carr A, et al. Reversibility of lipoatrophy in HIV-infected patients 2 years after switching from a thymidine analogue to abacavir: the MITOX Extension Study. *AIDS*. 2004;18:1029–1036.

173. McComsey GA, Ward DJ, Hessenthaler SM, et al. Improvement in lipoatrophy associated with highly active antiretroviral therapy in human immunodeficiency virus-infected patients switched from stavudine to abacavir or zidovudine: the results of the TARHEEL study. *Clin Infect Dis*. 2004;38:263–270.

174. Carr A, Workman C, Carey D, et al. No effect of rosiglitazone for treatment of HIV-1 lipoatrophy: randomised, double-blind, placebo-controlled trial. *Lancet*. 2004;363:429–438.

175. Slama L, Lanoy E, Valantin MA, et al. Effect of pioglitazone on HIV-1–related lipodystrophy: a randomized double-blind placebo-controlled trial (ANRS 113). *Antivir Ther*. 2008;13:67–76.

176. Hadigan C, Yawetz S, Thomas A, et al. Metabolic effects of rosiglitazone in HIV lipodystrophy: a randomized, controlled trial. *Ann Intern Med*. 2004;140:786–794.

177. Hsue PY, Giri K, Erickson S, et al. Clinical features of acute coronary syndromes in patients with human immunodeficiency virus infection. *Circulation*. 2004;109:316–319.

178. Matetzky S, Domingo M, Kar S, et al. Acute myocardial infarction in human immunodeficiency virus-infected patients. *Arch Intern Med*. 2003;163:457–460.

179. Boccara F, Cohen A, Di Angelantonio E, et al. Coronary artery bypass graft in HIV-infected patients: a multicenter case control study. *Curr HIV Res*. 2008;6:59–64.

180. Rerkpattanapipat P, Wongpraparut N, Jacobs LE, et al. Cardiac manifestations of acquired immunodeficiency syndrome. *Arch Intern Med*. 2000;160:602–608.

181. Currie PF, Jacob AJ, Foreman AR, et al. Heart muscle disease related to HIV infection: prognostic implications. *BMJ*. 1994;309:1605–1607.

182. Herskowitz A, Wu TC, Willoughby SB, et al. Myocarditis and cardiotropic viral infection associated with severe left

ventricular dysfunction in late-stage infection with human immunodeficiency virus. *J Am Coll Cardiol.* 1994;24:1025–1032.

183. Neumann T, Esser S, Potthoff A, et al. Prevalence and natural history of heart failure in outpatient HIV-infected subjects: rationale and design of the HIV-HEART study. *Eur J Med Res.* 2007;12:243–248.

184. Vellozzi C, Brooks JT, Bush TJ, et al. The study to understand the natural history of HIV and AIDS in the era of effective therapy (SUN Study). *Am J Epidemiol.* 2009;169:642–652.

185. Nayak G, Ferguson M, Tribble DR, et al. Cardiac diastolic dysfunction is prevalent in HIV-infected patients. *AIDS Patient Care STDS.* 2009;23:231–238.

186. Hsue PY, Farah H, Bolger A, et al. Diastolic dysfunction is common in asymptomatic HIV patients [abstr 979]. Program and Abstracts of the 16th Conference on Retroviruses and Opportunistic Infections, Montreal, PQ, Feb 8–11, 2009.

187. Grody WW, Cheng L, Lewis W. Infection of the heart by the human immunodeficiency virus. *Am J Cardiol.* 1990;66:203–206.

188. Raidel SM, Haase C, Jansen NR, et al. Targeted myocardial transgenic expression of HIV Tat causes cardiomyopathy and mitochondrial damage. *Am J Physiol Heart Circ Physiol.* 2002;282:H1672–H1678.

189. Sani MU. Myocardial disease in human immunodeficiency virus (HIV) infection: a review. *Wien Klin Wochenschr.* 2008;120:77–87.

190. Currie PF, Boon NA. Cardiac involvement in human immunodeficiency virus infection. *Q J Med.* 1993;86:751–753.

191. Herskowitz A, Willoughby SB, Baughman KL, et al. Cardiomyopathy associated with antiretroviral therapy in patients with HIV infection: a report of six cases. *Ann Intern Med.* 1992;116:311–313.

192. Tanuma J, Ishizaki A, Gatanaga H, et al. Dilated cardiomyopathy in an adult human immunodeficiency virus type 1–positive patient treated with a zidovudine-containing antiretroviral regimen. *Clin Infect Dis.* 2003;37:e109–e111.

193. Lewis W, Grupp IL, Grupp G, et al. Cardiac dysfunction occurs in the HIV-1 transgenic mouse treated with zidovudine. *Lab Invest*. 2000;80:187–197.
194. Carrillo-Jimenez R, Treadwell TL, Goldfine H, et al. Brain natriuretic peptide and HIV-related cardiomyopathy. *AIDS Read*. 2002;12:501–503, 508.
195. Cooper LT, Baughman KL, Feldman AM, et al. The role of endomyocardial biopsy in the management of cardiovascular disease: a scientific statement from the American Heart Association, the American College of Cardiology, and the European Society of Cardiology. Endorsed by the Heart Failure Society of America and the Heart Failure Association of the European Society of Cardiology. *J Am Coll Cardiol*. 2007;50:1914–1931.
196. Magnani JW, Dec GW. Myocarditis: current trends in diagnosis and treatment. *Circulation*. 2006;113:876–890.
197. Sitbon O, Lascoux-Combe C, Delfraissy JF, et al. Prevalence of HIV-related pulmonary arterial hypertension in the current antiretroviral therapy era. *Am J Respir Crit Care Med*. 2008; 177:108–113.
198. Speich R, Jenni R, Opravil M, et al. Primary pulmonary hypertension in HIV infection. *Chest*. 1991;100:1268–1271.
199. Lederman MM, Sereni D, Simonneau G, et al. Pulmonary arterial hypertension and its association with HIV infection: an overview. *AIDS*. 2008;22 Suppl 3:S1–S6.
200. Morse JH, Barst RJ, Itescu S, et al. Primary pulmonary hypertension in HIV infection: an outcome determined by particular HLA class II alleles. *Am J Respir Crit Care Med*. 1996;153:1299–1301.
201. Chin KM, Channick RN, Rubin LJ. Is methamphetamine use associated with idiopathic pulmonary arterial hypertension? *Chest*. 2006;130:1657–1663.
202. Runo JR, Loyd JE. Primary pulmonary hypertension. *Lancet*. 2003;361:1533–1544.
203. Diaz PT, King MA, Pacht ER, et al. Increased susceptibility to pulmonary emphysema among HIV-seropositive smokers. *Ann Intern Med*. 2000;132:369–372.

204. Klein SK, Slim EJ, de Kruif MD, et al. Is chronic HIV infection associated with venous thrombotic disease? A systematic review. *Neth J Med.* 2005;63:129–136.
205. Zuber JP, Calmy A, Evison JM, et al. Pulmonary arterial hypertension related to HIV infection: improved hemodynamics and survival associated with antiretroviral therapy. *Clin Infect Dis.* 2004;38:1178–1185.
206. Opravil M, Sereni D. Natural history of HIV-associated pulmonary arterial hypertension: trends in the HAART era. *AIDS.* 2008;22 Suppl 3:S35–S40.
207. Degano B, Yaici A, Le Pavec J, et al. Long-term effects of bosentan in patients with HIV-associated pulmonary arterial hypertension. *Eur Respir J.* 2009;33:92–98.
208. Sitbon O, Gressin V, Speich R, et al. Bosentan for the treatment of human immunodeficiency virus-associated pulmonary arterial hypertension. *Am J Respir Crit Care Med.* 2004;170:1212–1217.
209. Aguilar RV, Farber HW. Epoprostenol (prostacyclin) therapy in HIV-associated pulmonary hypertension. *Am J Respir Crit Care Med.* 2000;162:1846–1850.
210. Carlsen J, Kjeldsen K, Gerstoft J. Sildenafil as a successful treatment of otherwise fatal HIV-related pulmonary hypertension. *AIDS.* 2002;16:1568–1569.
211. Mehta NJ, Khan IA, Mehta RN, et al. HIV-Related pulmonary hypertension: analytic review of 131 cases. *Chest.* 2000;118:1133–1141.
212. Aschmann YZ, Kummer O, Linka A, et al. Pharmacokinetics and pharmacodynamics of sildenafil in a patient treated with human immunodeficiency virus protease inhibitors. *Ther Drug Monit.* 2008;30:130–134.
213. Merry C, Barry MG, Ryan M, et al. Interaction of sildenafil and indinavir when co-administered to HIV-positive patients. *AIDS.* 1999;13:F101–F107.
214. Chin KM, Rubin LJ. Pulmonary arterial hypertension. *J Am Coll Cardiol.* 2008;51:1527–1538.
215. Heidenreich PA, Eisenberg MJ, Kee LL, et al. Pericardial effusion in AIDS. Incidence and survival. *Circulation.* 1995;92:3229–3234.

216. Fisher SD, Lipshultz SE. Epidemiology of cardiovascular involvement in HIV disease and AIDS. *Ann N Y Acad Sci*. 2001;946:13–22.

217. Estok L, Wallach F. Cardiac tamponade in a patient with AIDS: a review of pericardial disease in patients with HIV infection. *Mt Sinai J Med*. 1998;65:33–39.

218. Imazio M, Trinchero R. Triage and management of acute pericarditis. *Int J Cardiol*. 2007;118:286–294.

219. Mayosi BM, Burgess LJ, Doubell AF. Tuberculous pericarditis. *Circulation*. 2005;112:3608–3616.

220. Manoff SB, Vlahov D, Herskowitz A, et al. Human immunodeficiency virus infection and infective endocarditis among injecting drug users. *Epidemiology*. 1996;7:566–570.

221. Nahass RG, Weinstein MP, Bartels J, et al. Infective endocarditis in intravenous drug users: a comparison of human immunodeficiency virus type 1–negative and -positive patients. *J Infect Dis*. 1990;162:967–970.

222. Gebo KA, Burkey MD, Lucas GM, et al. Incidence of, risk factors for, clinical presentation, and 1–year outcomes of infective endocarditis in an urban HIV cohort. *J Acquir Immune Defic Syndr*. 2006;43:426–432.

223. Ribera E, Miro JM, Cortes E, et al. Influence of human immunodeficiency virus 1 infection and degree of immunosuppression in the clinical characteristics and outcome of infective endocarditis in intravenous drug users. *Arch Intern Med*. 1998;158:2043–2050.

224. Stotka JL, Good CB, Downer WR, et al. Pericardial effusion and tamponade due to Kaposi's sarcoma in acquired immunodeficiency syndrome. *Chest*. 1989;95:1359–1361.

225. Steigman CK, Anderson DW, Macher AM, et al. Fatal cardiac tamponade in acquired immunodeficiency syndrome with epicardial Kaposi's sarcoma. *Am Heart J*. 1988;116:1105–1107.

226. Duong M, Dubois C, Buisson M, et al. Non-Hodgkin's lymphoma of the heart in patients infected with human immunodeficiency virus. *Clin Cardiol*. 1997;20:497–502.

227. Maric I, Washington S, Schwartz A, et al. Human herpesvirus-8–positive body cavity-based lymphoma involving the atria of the heart: a case report. *Cardiovasc Pathol.* 2002;11:244–247.

228. Tanaka PY, Atala MM, Pereira J, et al. Primary effusion lymphoma with cardiac involvement in HIV positive patient-complete response and long survival with chemotherapy and HAART. *J Clin Virol.* 2009;44:84–85.

229. Villa A, Foresti V, Confalonieri F. Autonomic neuropathy and prolongation of QT interval in human immunodeficiency virus infection. *Clin Auton Res.* 1995;5:48–52.

230. Eisenhauer MD, Eliasson AH, Taylor AJ, et al. Incidence of cardiac arrhythmias during intravenous pentamidine therapy in HIV-infected patients. *Chest.* 1994;105:389–395.

231. Gil M, Sala M, Anguera I, et al. QT prolongation and Torsades de Pointes in patients infected with human immunodeficiency virus and treated with methadone. *Am J Cardiol.* 2003;92:995–997.

232. Anson BD, Weaver JG, Ackerman MJ, et al. Blockade of HERG channels by HIV protease inhibitors. *Lancet.* 2005;365:682–686.

233. Charbit B, Rosier A, Bollens D, et al. Relationship between HIV protease inhibitors and QTc interval duration in HIV-infected patients: a cross-sectional study. *Br J Clin Pharmacol.* 2009;67:76–82.

234. Ly T, Ruiz ME. Prolonged QT interval and torsades de pointes associated with atazanavir therapy. *Clin Infect Dis.* 2007;44:e67–e68.

235. Gallagher DP, Kieran J, Sheehan G, et al. Ritonavir-boosted atazanavir, methadone, and ventricular tachycardia: 2 case reports. *Clin Infect Dis.* 2008;47:e36–e38.

236. Castillo R, Pedalino RP, El Sherif N, et al. Efavirenz-associated QT prolongation and Torsade de Pointes arrhythmia. *Ann Pharmacother.* 2002;36:1006–1008.

237. Kaletra (lopinavir/ritonavir) prescribing information, North Chicago, IL, Abbott Laboratories, April 2009 (package insert). 2009.

238. Busti AJ, Tsikouris JP, Peeters MJ, et al. A prospective evaluation of the effect of atazanavir on the QTc interval and QTc dispersion in HIV-positive patients. *HIV Med.* 2006;7:317–322.
239. Reyataz (atazanavir sulfate) prescribing information, Princeton, NJ, Bristol-Myers Squibb, April 2009 (package insert). 2009.
240. Gianotti N, Guffanti M, Galli L, et al. Electrocardiographic changes in HIV-infected, drug-experienced patients being treated with atazanavir. *AIDS.* 2007;21:1648–1651.
241. Mahnke L, Child M, Satin L, et al. Electrocardiographic changes in HIV-infected, drug experienced patients treated with atazanavir. *AIDS.* 2008;22:1698.